LAVENDER

LAVENDER

*Nature's Way to
Relaxation and Health*

PHILIPPA WARING

SOUVENIR PRESS

Typeset by FiSH Books
Printed and bound in Great Britain by the MPG Books Group

Some evidence has recently arisen to suggest that prolonged use by pre-adolescent boys of soaps and lotions containing lavender can initiate hormonal imbalances, possibly leading to symptoms such as the growth of breast-tissue. However, only three cases have been reported, and without a clear causal link being proven there may be no real risk. Nevertheless, be sure to seek immediate medical advice if such symptoms appear.

[Editor, 2010]

Contents

Author's Note

I have written this book to introduce readers to the remarkable qualities of lavender as a healer, relaxer, decoration and ingredient in home care and cooking. Its fascinating history goes back almost to the time when records began and helps to show just *why* the herb is held in such high esteem by people all over the world.

You will learn to grow and love lavender for all its aesthetic, healthful and delicious properties, and come to appreciate it in the garden, in the natural pharmacy and in the kitchen.

Philippa Waring
November 1996

PART 1

The Story of Lavender

Chapter 1
Nature's Great Restorer

To many people, lavender is just a typical plant of the cottage garden – fragrant and attractive to look at when in full summer bloom. Yet it is also a herb of hidden qualities, with a whole variety of uses to which it can be put in everyday life, health care and even the culinary arts. It is a constant source of surprise, too, as an accidental discovery by a French chemist in 1927 revealed: not only was a new element added to its list of properties, but a form of health treatment was born which now has followers all over the world.

That morning René-Maurice Gattefossé was working in his family's perfumery business, testing the essential oils of a number of plants used in the manufacture of the company's products. It was a study that had engaged his attention for several years and had already led to a number of advances in the techniques of distillation and blending. As the chemist worked at his bench a sudden explosion rocked the laboratory. Gattefossé fell back with a cry of pain, clutching at one of his hands which had been badly burned. Almost without thinking, as he later recounted, he thrust the injured hand into the nearest liquid, a container of pure lavender oil. The relief was almost instantaneous, and in the days that followed Gattefossé watched with mounting fascination and interest as his hand healed swiftly and cleanly, leaving no trace of a scar.

By the end of the week the conclusion was inescapable: lavender oil had the power to heal burns. The scientist in Gattefossé made him wonder if any of the other essential oils used in the business had similar healing powers which could make them as effective as, perhaps even more than, their chemical equivalents. He knew well enough from his study that these oils – odoriferous liquid components from aromatic plants, trees and grasses which had been extracted by steam distillation – were sometimes known as 'ethereal oils' because when they were left in the open air they evaporated without trace and as if by magic. But there was nothing supernatural about what he had stumbled upon, and Gattefossé was convinced that if he could substantiate the fact by further experimentation, a whole new branch of therapeutic treatment might be opened up. Later that year he wrote in what would become a landmark book:

> Doctors and chemists will be surprised at the range of odoriferous substances which may be used medically and at the great variety of their chemical functions. Beside the antiseptic and antimicrobial properties of which use is currently made, the essential oils are also antitoxic and antiviral, they have a powerful energising effect and possess an undeniable cicatrising property. In the future their role will be even greater.

Gattefossé's words could hardly have been more prophetic. Nor was his contribution quite finished, because in order to describe this use to which essential oils might be put in health care he coined the term 'aromatherapy', which he also used as the title for his book, published the following year. Today, anyone who practises this branch of complementary medicine should be aware of the debt they owe to the humble lavender plant.

It is probably true to say that most modern gardens of any size contain at least one lavender bush. Some, like my grandmother's, have a whole range of different varieties: I remember that hers looked especially beautiful in the summer months with their purple, blue and pink flowers scenting the garden with their unique, sweet fragrance. The old lady, who died when well into her eighties, had a special fondness for the herb and throughout her home the evidence was there for all to see.

In the winter, for example, she took full advantage of her summer crop of lavender to perfume her little cottage with bunches of the flowers that hung in posies in a number of the rooms. She also used the dried flowers in embroidered lavender bags which kept her cupboards and drawers sweet-smelling and free of moths and other insects. In the bathroom cabinet she had a small, dark blue bottle marked 'Lavender Oil' which she used for emergencies. When, one day, I was stung by a wasp, a couple of drops which she administered to my swollen arm quickly brought relief and stopped my tears. She made up lavender water to cool and refresh herself on hot days, and dab on the neck and hem of her dress so that she seemed to waft through life trailing an unmistakable aroma. When she kissed me, the fragrance of lavender stayed in my nostrils for hours afterwards.

My grandmother also brewed lavender tea which she said was good for headaches and stopped you from worrying, and that would make you live longer. She used cooking apples and lavender to make jars of jelly conserve which tasted absolutely delicious on fresh bread or toast. Occasionally, I remember, she would even hum a little rhyme as she cleaned the house:

> Velvet gown and dainty fur
> Should be laid in lavender,
> For its sweetness drives away
> Fretting moths of silver grey.

The mere aroma of lavender, she once confided to me as we sat in her kitchen on a bleak winter morning, provided her with a constant reminder of the drowsy, fragrant days of summer. Not surprisingly, it was from her that I first began to learn some of the secrets of this extraordinary plant and its remarkable properties, as healer, household aid and cookery ingredient. Those properties have made it a boon to mankind since the days of Ancient Rome.

The lavender plant belongs to the family Labiatae and is of the genus *Lavandula*, indicating that the flowers are tubular and lipped, although they vary in shape and appearance. The range of its varieties is enormous: some types are no more than little shrubs while others form tall and impressive growths as much as five feet high. Because of this, lavender may be grown in solitary splendour, in small groups, or as a hedge to border the garden.

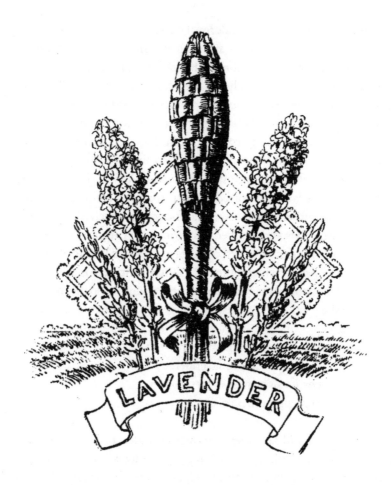

The lavender plant has inspired and rewarded centuries
of human ingenuity (*Pip Miller*).

The plant is a xerophyte, which means that it is especially adept at
thriving in dry conditions. The coarse, greyish leaves are the
giveaway of this quality – the greyness actually being a mass of tiny
white hairs which are there to hold moisture within the plant. In an
article in *The Times* about the climatic changes taking place in

Britain, with the country becoming more Mediterranean, it was reported that tests carried out by the Henry Doubleday Research Association in its gardens at Ryton near Coventry and Yalding near Maidstone, Kent, had revealed that lavender was 'high on the list of plants that can survive drought and still flower plentifully'. This is because it has evolved a strategy to deal with the sun and the consequent risk of desiccation. In addition it has an extensive root system which can go as deep as 75 cm (2ft 6ins).

Originally, of course, lavender grew only in the wild, and it was from its wild form that mankind first began to learn of its herbal benefits. Subsequent interbreeding of the species has produced plants with colours ranging from deepest purple through the traditional 'lavender' to the palest shades of pink and white, and with many different types of leaf shape and texture.

Although for a time in recent years lavender was considered old-fashioned, with a fragrance that harked back to Victorian times (as exemplified by the term 'lavender and old lace'), it is now enjoying a new wave of popularity, not just as a perfume but also as a flavouring and decoration. Cultivation and hybridisation are also constantly producing new varieties with different benefits.

England and France are probably the two countries most readily associated with the cultivation of lavender – in the UK in Norfolk and the Cotswolds, and across the Channel mainly between Orange and Grasse – but it is also grown in quite a number of other countries. Although I would not claim the list to be definitive, I know that it is to be found in Germany, Holland, Belgium, Spain, Portugal, Italy, Hungary, Bulgaria, Romania, Algeria, Morocco and Turkey, as well as the United States, Canada, Russia, China, Japan and Australia. Indeed, during the course of writing this book I found myself consulting dictionaries of several different languages to find the common name of the herb in each country. Those which remain fixed in my mind include *Lavande* (France), *Lavanda* (Italy), *Lavendel* (Germany), *Lavendel* (Holland), *Espliego* (Spain) and, most curious of all, *Alfazema* in Portugal.

Lavender is still found growing wild in many parts of the Mediterranean region on dry, warm slopes, as far east as Greece, and it can be spotted sporadically as high up as the tree limit – about 1,707 metres (5,600 feet) – on some mountains like the Maritime Alps. In Germany there is even an area between Bingen and Kreuznach where it is so widespread that the local people call the region the 'Lavender Mountain'.

One cannot help wondering if this place was a source of inspiration for the expression 'being in lavender' as opposed to the more famous term which refers to clover. In one of the early editions of that wonderful reference book, *Dictionary of Phrase and Fable*, compiled by the admirable Ebenezer Cobham Brewer almost 150 years ago, I found this entry: '*Laid up in lavender*, i.e. taken great care of, laid away, as women put things away in lavender to keep off moths. Things in pawn, or persons in hiding, are said to be in lavender.'

The properties of lavender in either its essential oil form or as dried flowers are such that over the years it has been prescribed for all manner of ailments – some of these suggestions being vaguely practical while the rest are outlandish, to say the least. For example, I have found it recommended for the bite of a mad dog, to exorcise ghosts and prevent pregnancy, and even to cure baldness! More realistic is the entry in that *vade mecum* of natural medicine, Nicholas Culpeper's *Complete Herbal*, which I referred to at an early point in my research. A nineteenth-century edition comments:

Lavender is of special good use for all the griefs and pains of the head and brains that proceed of a cold cause, as the apoplexy, falling sickness, the sluggish malady, cramps, convulsions, palsies and often faintings. It strengtheneth the stomach, and freeth the liver and spleen from obstructions, provoketh women's courses and expelleth the child and afterbirth. The flowers of lavender, steeped in wine, helpeth them that are troubled with the wind, or colic, if the places be bathed therewith. A decoction made with flowers of Lavender, Horehound, Fennel and Asparagus roots, with a little cinnamon, is very profitably used to help the falling sickness, and the giddiness or turning of the brain. To gargle the mouth with the decoction thereof is good against the toothache. Two spoonfuls of the distilled water of the flowers taken, helpeth them that have lost their voice, as also the tremblings and passions of the heart, and faintings and swoonings, not only being drunk, but applied to the temples, or the nostrils to be smelt into. But it is not safe to use it where the body is repleat with blood and humours, because of the hot and subtle spirits wherewith it is possessed. The oil used with the Oil of Spike is of a fierce and piercing quality, and ought to be carefully used, a very few drops being sufficient for inward or outward maladies.

Research into the lavender plant has progressed a long way since Culpeper wrote those lines in about 1653; while many of his cures are still relevant in more modern versions, we now know a lot more about the herb, although the central mystery of just *why* it does what it does still eludes researchers. Henry Head, the managing director of Norfolk Lavender at Heacham, who has been very helpful to me in the writing of this book, explained, 'It is precisely because we are *not* sure which are the active ingredients in lavender that are said to help in stress relief, skin care and the like, that we are instituting research.'

The flowers of the lavender contain approximately 12 per cent tannin as well as up to 3 per cent ethereal oils (*oleum lavandulae*). The principal constituents of the oils are linalyl and geranyl esters, geranial, linalool and a little coumarin. (Essential oils in general have complex molecular structures and may contain up to several hundred different natural chemicals which, when the oils are mixed in appropriate blends, are said to have tremendous therapeutic potential.)

Because the glands or calyx containing the oil are easily accessible at the base of each floret, extracting it is most efficiently achieved by distillation. In this process, the flowers are packed tightly into a still and steam is forced through them. The heat causes the glands to burst open and the oil mixes with the steam. A cooling process then returns the vapours to their liquid state and the pale yellow lavender oil separates from the water and can be collected. I shall be describing this process more fully later in the book.

However, since most people are likely to buy lavender oil ready-bottled, this is perhaps a suitable point at which to offer a few words of advice *before* anyone gets too carried away with the idea of putting it to work in any of the different uses discussed in the following pages:

1   Only buy lavender oil of the highest quality from a reputable supplier (there are already quite a number of cheaper and inferior brands creeping onto the market). Ensure that it is sold in a small brown glass bottle and that the label is marked with the words 'Pure Essential Oil' and the precise amount of the contents.

2   Store the oil (or any blend of essential oils that you have prepared from instructions) in a cool, dark place, as heat, light and air can spoil its healing properties – 18°C (65°F) is ideal. And do make sure that the bottle top is *always* tightly secured.

3   Essential oils are extremely concentrated and should always be used carefully. Most must be diluted in a carrier oil for such uses as skin care and massage.

4   In most instances, only a few drops of lavender oil should be used at any one time, and these should be dispensed by an eye-dropper or pipette. Keep the bottle away from the reach of small children!

5   If lavender oil is correctly stored it will keep for several years, but if it is mixed with other oils these should not be used after nine months.

Lavender can be used in various medical and therapeutic ways in compresses and lotions, in baths, oil burners or neat as an instant form of first aid. Its qualities may be categorised as analgesic (relieving pain), antidepressant, anti-inflammatory, antiseptic, anti-spasmodic, carminative (relieving flatulence), cicatrisant (healing of wounds), deodorant, diuretic, emmenagogue (stimulating blood flow in the pelvic area and uterus), expectorant, hypotensive, nervine (soothing the nerves) and sedative. No mean list, and the problems which it can help to combat are these:

- *Breathing.* Because lavender is an antiseptic it can kill micro-organisms, and it is also an expectorant which facilitates the break-up of catarrh. It can help fight colds, throat infections, coughs, sinusitis and flu.

- *Circulation.* The oil is a sedative and hypotensive and can reduce high blood pressure and palpitations. As a diuretic, lavender is said to have a particular affinity with the kidneys and promotes the flow of urine.

- *Deodorant.* The antiseptic and cleansing qualities fight sweat while the fragrance of lavender combats body odour. Preparations with lavender can be used by both men and women.

- *Digestion.* Use of lavender, which is a carminative and cleanser, will help indigestion, flatulence and nausea and alleviate bad breath and toothache.

- *Emotion.* With its antidepressant and sedative qualities, lavender can help to lift depression, ease stress and anxiety, and is useful in overcoming headaches, migraine and insomnia. The nervine in it is a tonic for nervous disorders.

- *Gynaecological.* Lavender has a calming influence, can ease premenstrual and menopausal symptoms, and is helpful in promoting menstrual regularity and curing thrush. Because it is a mild emmenagogue which can induce or stimulate the menstrual flow, **it should be avoided for the first seven months of pregnancy**.

- *Insomnia.* The sedative quality of lavender can induce sleep and ease problems of insomnia, restlessness and agitation, particularly in the old with whom it is said to have fewer side-effects than prescribed drugs.

- *Muscular.* As an analgesic, anti-inflammatory and anti-spasmodic, the oil is good for muscular aches, pains, sprains, rheumatism spasms and cramp.

- *Skin.* Because lavender is an antiseptic, anti-inflammatory and a cicatrisant, it promotes the formation of scar tissue and can ease burns, insect bites and sunburn, as well as clearing up acne, boils, eczema and dandruff.

Throughout my research for this book, I have been constantly surprised at the versatility of the plant, the many uses to which it can be put, and the enormous pleasure it can give to gardeners, herbalists and cooks – not to mention the increasing amount of attention it has been getting in the British national press as its qualities have come under discussion.

In September 1995, for example, *The Observer* revealed that lavender oil was being used as part of a course of aromatherapy, funded by Age Concern and the Kingston and Richmond Health Authority, to ease the symptoms of Alzheimer's disease in a group of 50 elderly people in the district. During a six-month period regular massage with essential oils had worked wonders in cutting back their dependence on medication and had boosted their general health, mobility and sense of well-being. Several reported that their limbs were less painful, they were less depressed and were sleeping a great deal better. 'The smell of lavender oil is especially lovely,' one woman declared, 'and it's even cleared up my chest.'

Two months later, in a major article on job-related stress in *The Mail on Sunday*, alternative practitioner Hamida Bellenie stated that, for instant relief, 'people should keep a small bottle of famous stress-beaters such as lavender essential oil on their desks and use them when the going gets tough.' (The Japanese, I am told, have take this idea a step further: in some buildings lavender-scented air is being pumped directly into offices via the air-conditioning in order to beat stress and help maintain concentration.)

A few weeks later the *Daily Mail* devoted a whole page to what it called 'the scented soothers from nature's own medicine chest'. In the course of this it said that lavender, 'often used in de-stressing treatments, also acts as a great tonic for tired skin – boosting lymphatic circulation while temporarily firming and tightening the surface cells.' Then, in March 1996, *The Independent on Sunday* went even further, declaring that 'lavender oil is said by aromatherapists to be the most relaxing essence available to the public.'

The media have also become increasingly interested in the research being conducted in scientific establishments like Warwick University, into the specific effects of certain essential oils on the mind and central nervous system. Yet with all the technical wizardry of EEC machines and the like, they have actually only been able to confirm what many have known about lavender for centuries – that it has a predominantly sedative and antidepressant effect. What is perhaps more enlightening is the suggestion coming from one or two experts in the field of alternative medicine, that what makes flower oil remedies work may be the plant's own energy which functions on a 'vibrational' level within the body. However, this theory is admittedly difficult to prove: a plant's energy cannot be detected in the way that pain-killing ingredients can.

In the United States it is being suggested that lavender's rising popularity is due to a combination of its scent and the effect it has upon the *personality* of people. Annette Green of the charmingly named Fragrance Foundation has been quoted as saying, 'The future of fragrance lies with aromachology, the science of creating fragrant products which have a tangible effect on the psyche as well as smelling great.'

What might almost be described as an attempt to put this into effect was the launch in Paris in July 1996 of a lavender-based scent, 'A Year in Provence', inspired by the best-selling books of Peter Mayle about his life in that beautiful area of France. The perfumer behind the product, Agnes Costa, explained, 'We wanted to re-create the smell of clean white linen drying in the Provençal sunshine surrounded by fields of lavender.' The cologne, which contains a mixture of lavender and white musk, is intended for both men and women.

Although certain perfume manufacturers, scientists and others in the field of commerce may try to present lavender as the new fashion of the moment, it has had its admirers for centuries. In the past, a great many men and women have realised the potential of the plant and added to our store of knowledge – people like the Head family who run Norfolk Lavender in Heacham (of which more later); Joan Head (no relation) of Clipston-on-the-Wolds near Keyworth, Nottinghamshire, who grows lavender and publishes a magazine devoted to the plant, *The Lavender Bag*; David and Elizabeth Christie of Jersey Lavender with their impressive gardens full of different varieties; and Natalie Hodgson who operated the only pick-your-own lavender farm in the country at Astley Abbotts near Bridgnorth in Shropshire. Started in 1989, Mrs Hodgson's lavender fields now attract thousands of visitors each year, who are provided with scissors and allowed to cut as much as they like. What is left at the end of August is sold for distilling into essential oil.

Lavender, as the reader will discover, is a hardy, fragrant and valuable plant with a colourful history and almost limitless potential. But it also offers a unique and intensely personal experience. If you want to know what I mean, just smell the flowers when they are in bloom, or rub some of the dried heads between your fingers, or just tip a few drops of the oil into your bath. The aroma and feeling of relaxation that will envelop you are living proof of the spell lavender has woven over mankind since time immemorial.

Chapter 2
Lavender in Folklore and History

A very old European tradition maintains that the first lavender bush grew in the Garden of Eden and that Adam and Eve brought a sprig of the fragrant plant with them when they were expelled from their idyllic existence. Fable or not, there is evidence that as long ago as 4000 BC the herb was being used by people in the East, who had devised methods of pressing, boiling and macerating essences from its flowers. Because the process was laborious and the amounts of oil extracted small, these products were invariably reserved exclusively for the use of kings and queens and their favourite courtiers and priests.

The great antiquity of lavender is evident in the accounts of the *Nardus stricta* and *Nardus indica* by very early writers who also comment on its importance (*nardus* was the Latin word for lavender, from the Greek *nard*). The Ancient Egyptians were devotees of perfumes and massage oils and were among the first to open up trade in such things with other civilisations. It was in Egypt that lavender enjoyed its first little taste of notoriety, because rumour had it that the asp which killed Queen Cleopatra had been found under a lavender bush! The pharaoh Tutankhamun was laid in his tomb with a perfume jar of lavender at his side.

The Greeks held the plant in high esteem, too, and it was one of their writers, Pedanius Dioscorides, whom I mentioned in Chapter Seven, who was responsible for noting the use of lavender in medicine during the first century AD. The Romans, if anything, valued the herb even more highly than their neighbours and there is evidence of this in two of the works by the great Latin poet Virgil, the *Eclogues* and the *Georgics*. In these he shows that his countrymen were pioneers in what was almost an industry in the preparation of oils and perfumes.

Lavender was used to scent the public baths and those of the wealthier and more important members of Roman society. The notorious Emperor Caligula, for instance, believed that aromatic baths of the herb would restore his vitality after he had become run down by sexual excess. The oil from the plant was also used by the Romans to massage and heal the skin, and as an insecticide to repel fleas, mosquitoes, lice and other household pests. No self-respecting householder would have a bed without its special holders of dried lavender to keep it free of bedbugs, and one of the most popular of all Roman perfumes, *nardinum*, was made of lavender, myrrh and ground-up lilies. Such was the honour in which lavender was held in Roman society that it was also frequently burnt in honour of the gods.

It seems likely that it was the Romans who first introduced lavender to Britain, although the possibility cannot be ruled out that the plant, with its ability to grow in stony soil and thrive in a dry climate, was already established in some sunny corners of the land. Be that as it may, the all-conquering Roman troops certainly brought lavender with them to be used by injured and battle-weary soldiers, and were the first to plant it for harvesting and processing. Sadly, after the Romans left these islands and Britain was over-run by the Anglo-Saxon invaders, many of the secrets of lavender were forgotten.

There are, of course, several references to lavender in the Bible. The Queen of Sheba is said to have offered King Solomon 'myrrh, frankincense and spike' (Indian spike was an early name for lavender) and it was a lavender oil that Judith rubbed all over her body before setting off to seduce and murder Holofernes, the Assyrian commander. A Christian legend says that originally lavender had no scent – until, that is, the Virgin Mary dried the swaddling clothes of the infant Jesus on it: ever since it has had its 'heavenly' scent.

During medieval times it was the religious establishments of Europe which appreciated the value of lavender. Monks across the length and breadth of the continent grew a whole variety of herbs in their gardens for use in both cooking and medicine, and documents of the period indicate that lavender was one of the most commonly grown plants. It is claimed that in the twelfth century the Benedictine Abbess Hildegard, whose priory was at Bingen on the Rhine, was the first to distil lavender water in the form we recognise today.

There is also evidence of its use in a different way in France during this period. Here the flowers were strewn on the floors to mask household smells, as well as in the doorways leading to the stinking, insanitary streets outside. A legend that the glove-makers of Grasse, who used lavender oil to scent their leather, seemed always to avoid the ravages of the plague spurred many other people in France to carry lavender on their person. In the fourteenth century Charles VI, who as we will see liked to relax on white satin cushions stuffed with lavender, had a special preparation made up for him which was said to be good for 'annointing the fevered brow' and contained dried lavender and rosemary flowers plus cloves, nutmeg, mace, cardamom, cinnamon and a few rose petals all mixed in a quart of aquavita. Sounds to me like a rather strange cure for a hangover!

It was around this time that judges began to carry posies containing lavender (among other herbs) to ward off the noxious smells of the prisoners who were brought before them in the courts. Known as 'tussie-mussies', they were believed to be a protection against illness, and many of the great and good would carry them around under the impression that the sweet scent would counteract the perils of the disease-ridden streets and drains. This tradition – famously employed by the legendary eighteenth-century 'blind beak', Sir John Fielding, the Bow Street magistrate and detective who organised the first force of thief-takers to which his court gave its name – continued to be used by a number of assize judges until the last century, and it lingers on in the Maundy Thursday ceremony, when the British monarch carries a posy while distributing coins to the poor.

According to the sixteenth-century *Hortus Britannicus*, lavender was first cultivated as a crop in England in 1568, but where the unknown compilers got their facts for such a specific date is puzzling. The records of Melton Priory in Leicestershire show that lavender had been one of the crops in the herb garden there since as early as the year 1301! Little further mention of it is made for the next two hundred years, however, until the appearance of the earliest known really original work on gardening, a treatise in verse, *A Feate of Gardening*, by 'Mayster Ion Gardener'. A copy of this unique work still exists in the library of Trinity College, Cambridge, and is believed to have been written about 1440, although the poem itself is probably of an even earlier date. Of 'Ion' – or John – very little is known beyond the fact that he was from Kent and may well have been a professional gardener. In this thoroughly practical work, lavender is mentioned under several headings including 'Herbys necessary for a garden by letter' and 'Also of the same Herbes for a Salade'.

In the sixteenth century the herbalist William Turner praised lavender as 'a comfort to the braine' – advice that Queen Elizabeth I may well have taken because she is reputed to have drunk as many as ten cups of lavender tea per day to relieve her migraines. These pains were obviously not bad enough to spoil her sweet tooth, because Elizabeth is also said to have been very fond of lavender conserve made by dipping the flowers of the plant into lashings of sugar. Just how keen the Queen was to have a constant supply of lavender may be judged from the fact that she had in her employ a waiting-woman on a fixed salary, whose job it was to have flowers always in readiness, especially for strewing. As late as 1713 there is evidence that this office was still extant, according to a letter in the State Archives addressed to Alice Blizard who held the post of 'herbe strewer to Her Majesty the Queen'.

If Queen Elizabeth I may be counted as one of the first royal promoters of the value of lavender, Edward VI, the only son of Henry VIII by his third queen, Jane Seymour, actually employed a laundryman who was known as the 'lavender man'. According to Edward's court manual, The Black Book, the man was authorised to procure 'sufficient whyte soap tenderly to wasshe the stuffe from the King's propyr person'. His laundry quarters were apparently famous for the number of lavender bunches that hung around the walls and the fact that all the monarch's linen was stored with lavender bags.

William Shakespeare was one of a number of writers who have provided us with clues to the increasing use of lavender at this time. Lines about lavender can be found in several of his works, including his mention of herbs 'smelling as sweet at Bucklersbury in simpling time', a reference to the London herb market of Tudor days; or, more famously still, in *The Winter's Tale*:

> Here's flowers for you;
> Hot lavender, mints, savory, marjoram,
> The marigold, that goes to bed wi' the sun,
> And with him rises weeping.

One of Shakespeare's contemporaries, Robert Greene, a dramatist from Norwich whose romance *Pandosto* is said to have supplied the bard with ideas for the plot of *The Winter's Tale*, was obviously also interested in the traditions surrounding lavender, and suggests in a passage in his work *Quips* that it was then regarded in some quarters as an emblem of cuckoldom. 'There was loyal lavender,' he wrote, 'but that was full of cuckowspittes, to show that women's light thoughts make their husbands heavy heads.'

Another writer of the period, the pastoral poet Michael Drayton of Warwickshire, famous for his *Poly-olbion* and volume of eclogues, *The Shepherd's Garland*, mentions the use of the plant in the pleasant custom observed by young girls of sending lavender garlands to their lovers as signs of affection:

> He from his lasse him lavender hath sent,
> Shewing her love and doth requittal crave,
> Him rosemary his sweet-heart, whose intent
> Is that, he her should in remembrance have.

In more everyday use, lavender was employed in the house to keep linen fresh and free from moths; mixed with beeswax to polish furniture; to scent tobacco and snuff; and mixed with charcoal for cleaning the teeth. Among country people, it was held to be good for colds. Sufferers either bathed their temples with lavender water or took fresh sprigs of the plant and put them into a quilted cap to be worn on the head. In some districts, lavender was used as a folk remedy for epilepsy and was held to be good for 'colic, stomach cramps, dropsy, vapours and faintness'.

Lavender even found its place in the armoury of charms devised to combat superstition. For centuries, the Devil had been believed to interfere in the lives of men and women, and those who feared that Old Nick might come by night to seize them from their beds thought they would be safe if they hung a cross made of lavender flowers on the front door. This means of protection is very similar to that used by people in Hungary, Romania and Transylvania, who believed a garland of garlic would keep them safe from vampires. In Ireland, any young girl who wore a garter made from lavender was said to be safe from the spells of witches. More curious still, in 1578 Francis Lyte wrote in his *Dodoens* that 'lavender is of two sorts, male and female', while a century later John Hale in *Primitive Origins of Man* (1677) declared that 'the seeds of lavender kept a little warm and moist *will turn into moths*' [my italics].

The year 1629 saw the publication of another milestone in gardening literature, in which the qualities of lavender were extolled in glowing terms: *Paradisi in Sole, Paradisus Terrestris; or, A Garden of all Sorts of Pleasant Flowers with a Kitchen Garden by John Parkinson*. The title, a play upon the author's name, 'Park-in-Sun's Earthly Paradise', displayed all the author's love for plants and herbs, which he had developed during his years as an apothecary and botanist in London where he tended a much-admired garden. He dedicated the work to Queen Henrietta Maria, the mother of Charles II, who had an excellent garden in Wimbledon where she grew numerous varieties of lavender to satisfy her partiality for lavender wine and lavender conserve. Just what value John Parkinson put on lavender may be judged by this typical sentence from his *Paradisi*: 'Lavender is almost wholly spent with us, for to perfume linnen, apparrell, gloves, leather & the dryed flowers to comfort and dry up the moisture of a cold braine.'

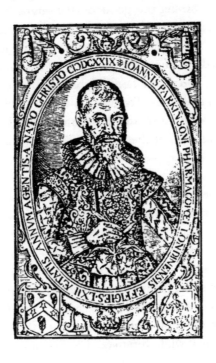

John Parkinson (from the title page of his *Paradisi in Sole, Paradisus Terrestris*).

Nell Gwyn, the famous mistress of Charles II, was born in humble circumstances in Hereford, and grew up with a love of lavender as well as the oranges she sold in London, which led to her introduction to the King. She is said to have exchanged sachets of lavender with Charles as Christmas presents. Lavender was put to a quite different use during the Great Plague of 1665. Because of its reputation as a curative, wealthy Londoners bought up all the supplies of the plant they could obtain, to burn and thus cleanse the air. Curiously, a group of thieves caught in the act of robbing the homes of plague victims said they had covered themselves with lavender water as a protection against the disease. The fact that they had survived sent the reputation of lavender even higher!

Such tales did nothing but good for the young lavender-sellers who crowded the streets of London with their cries which, for generations, were a notable feature of everyday city life. They were first immortalised in *The Cryes of the City of London* by Pierce Tempest in 1688, and, most famously of all, in Henry Mayhew's *London Labour and London Poor*, which began publication in the *Morning Chronicle* in 1849 and has gone through innumerable editions ever since. Two of the most familiar lavender-sellers' cries were these:

> Here's fine lavender for your cloaths,
> Come buy my fine lavender!

Or alternatively:

> Lavender, sweet blooming lavender,
> Six bunches a penny today.
> Lavender, sweet blooming lavender,
> Ladies, buy it while you may.

The last line took on an added significance during the years of pestilence and fever, and some of the sellers were able to make a good living – so long as their supplies from farms in Surrey, Hertfordshire and Kent did not run out. One of the most famous lavender-sellers of the Stuart period was 'Nosegay Fan' Barton who worked the area of Drury Lane and was said, during hard times, to be willing to sell her pretty body to any wealthy man-about-town who wanted a little more than one of her posies.

An eighteenth-century Scottish quack who tried to cash in on the health-giving reputation of lavender was 'Doctor' James Graham who set up 'Temples of Health and Hymen' in London, where he prescribed a variety of remedies to his gullible patients. Although he had studied medicine in Glasgow, Graham never graduated but still managed to gain many wealthy and influential clients, among them the Prince of Wales and the Duchess of Devonshire. In 1780 he revealed his most amazing creation, 'The Celestial Bed', which, he claimed, would ensure its occupants a better love life. The bed was said to be perfumed with 'Arabian spices in the style of those of the seraglio of the Grand Turk'. What the mattress actually contained was a mixture of lavender flowers, lemon balm and rose petals, plus 'the hairs from the tails of full-blooded black stallions to ensure virility'.

It was in France, where itinerant distillers had for years travelled with their mobile stills to wherever lavender was harvested, that a remarkable development took place in 1826. A chemist named Joseph Nicephore Niepce succeeded in producing the first 'photograph' on metal by using a mixture of lavender and bitumen of Judaea which changes its solubility in the herb when exposed to light. His later work with Louis Daguerre resulted in the 'daguerrotype' and, ultimately, modern photography. Today, lavender's contribution in the birth of the cinema is commemorated in the slang term 'lavender', often heard in film studios and processing laboratories. The great film director Cecil B. De Mille explained the use of the term in 1936: 'A "lavender" is a print made from a negative on lavender stock, which is a weak print from a weak negative, because lavender negatives are only copies of the film originally exposed in the camera and are therefore not as sharp.'

The Victorian era was another high spot in the history of lavender. Queen Victoria was a great user of lavender water, essential oils and a number of perfumes which contained the herb; indeed, she had her own special supplier, Sarah Sprules, who basked in the title 'Purveyor of Lavender Essence to Her Majesty the Queen', and as a result was much sought after by fashionable ladies in society. Lavender water was particularly popular with those women who had to follow their soldier and statesmen husbands to the far corners of the earth. They could, however, take special comfort from the words of Charles McIntosh in his *Book of the Garden*, published in 1855, in which he wrote, 'The lavender-water made of home-grown flowers is considered superior to that imported from France.' This widespread familiarity with the product came in for a little comic treatment by that great writer of nonsense verse, Edward Lear. Lear, who was himself an inveterate traveller, wrote in 'The Pobble Who Has No Toes':

> And his Aunt Jobiska made him drink,
> Lavender water tinged with pink,
> For she said, 'The world in general knows,
> There's nothing so good for a Pobble's toes!'

The use of lavender by heroines was a familiar theme in Victorian literature, too, and in 1902 the appearance of a book entitled *Lavender and Old Lace*, by the romantic novelist Myrtle Reed, added a new expression to the English language. Since then, according to the *Oxford English Dictionary*, the title of Miss Reed's story has been used 'to describe a gentle and old-fashioned style of novel'. In 1938 the book was adapted for the London stage by Rose Warner and ran for almost two years.

Lavender was put to a more serious use during World War One, when the terrible toll of men in the trenches of France made it impossible for the doctors and medical orderlies to keep enough supplies of the normal medicines to meet demand. In dire need, they turned to lavender and, inspired to a considerable degree by the early experimental work of René-Maurice Gattefossé, used the plant's essential oil as an antiseptic swab for war wounds. The oil was applied on sphagnum moss as a dressing and there is little doubt that it saved the limbs of many badly injured soldiers.

In the Thirties the demand for lavender fell, due mainly to the enormous increase in the number of proprietary domestic cleaners which came on the market, and the grandiloquent claims made by some medical manufacturers for the curative powers of their drugs. Now, thanks to the renewed interest in herbal medicines and the ever-increasing acceptance of aromatherapy, lavender is once again playing its time-honoured and important role in the first aid cabinets, homes and kitchens of people all over the world.

Chapter 3
The Essence of Lavender

At first glance it appears almost as if the sea has rolled in from the Wash onto the wild and unspoilt North Norfolk coast, and swathed the sandy countryside in gently rolling waves of purple-blue. On closer inspection, the undulations lying beside the A149 King's Lynn-to-Hunstanton road, near the village of Heacham, turn out to be row upon row of lavender, the flowers vivid in the bright sunlight of a summer morning. In the midst of this sea of colour – the unmistakable fragrance of the plant wafting on the summer breeze – a lavender cutter, manned by three men, manoeuvres steadily up and down the rows, bringing in the harvest.

Heacham is the home of English lavender, the only full-scale lavender farm in the country, where the herb has now been cultivated for more than sixty years. From the initial planting in 1932 of 13,000 plants spread over 2.4 hectares (six acres), carried out by three men and a boy, the business now covers over 40 hectares (100 acres) – half of which are at Sandringham, one of the homes of the Royal Family – and generates around 150 tons of lavender to be harvested each year in July and August. Henry Head, the hard-working boss of the family-run enterprise, reckoned that if all the lavender bushes were planted in one long row it would stretch for 193 kilometres (120 miles) – or from the Wash to the centre of London.

The reasons for growing lavender here are two-fold: the low annual rainfall of 45–48 cm (18–19 inches), and the light, sandy soil which is also quite chalky, with a pH of between seven and eight, ideal for the herb. Norfolk Lavender grow mainly varieties of the *L. angustifolia* species which is renowned for the quality of its oil and the rich, dark purple flowers which are perfect for pot-pourri and floral decorations.

The area is famous not only for its lavender, however. It was a Heacham man, John Rolfe, an English settler in America in the early years of the seventeenth century, who introduced tobacco planting to Virginia and in 1613 married the Native American princess Pocahontas and brought her back to his ancestral home in Heacham. Pocahontas, who famously saved the life of Captain John Smith from the tomahawks of her father Powhatan's braves, has recently been the subject of a hugely successful if rather romanticised Walt Disney cartoon film. In the village she enjoys a more modest if enduring fame: there is an alabaster tablet to her memory in the thirteenth-century church of St Mary, showing her wearing richly ornate clothing from the reign of James I, complete with a high hat and fan of three feathers. She also appears in the same dress on the village sign. This sign, which appropriately features bunches of lavender, stands immediately opposite the entrance to Caley Mill, the heart of the Norfolk Lavender business, where the harvest of flowers is brought from the fields for processing into essential oil or, alternatively, for drying. It is here, too, that the National Collection of lavenders is being developed, currently with over 100 species and cultivars and increasing in numbers all the time (see Chapter Four).

The history of Norfolk Lavender represents the realisation of the dream of one man, Linn Chilvers, whose signature is to be found on every product that bears the company's label. It is a story interestingly associated with the Royal Family who have been admirers of the virtues of lavender for many years. Queen Victoria, for example, used to sprinkle lavender on her handkerchiefs and insisted on lavender jelly on her roast mutton, while both the Queen and the Duke of Edinburgh are said to enjoy the invigorating rides through the lavender fields. In 1874 Linn Chilvers' father started a nursery garden and florist's business in Heacham and Hunstanton, and such was his skill that he won a Royal Warrant to supply plants to Queen Alexandra, the wife of King Edward VII, for the Sandringham gardens. Linn shared his father's interest in lavender which grew easily on the well-drained, alkaline soil of the area, with its exceptional exposure to sunlight – Norfolk has more sun than many others parts of England; he also nursed a desire to use it as the basis for a commercial venture.

In the years up to and following World War One the focus of the lavender industry had been farther south, around Mitcham in Surrey, where for almost two hundred years the firm of Potter and Moore had been the leading distillers and manufacturers of commercial products emanating from the plant. Cultivating their crops in fields in Mitcham and the surrounding districts of Carshalton and Wallington, they had made 'Mitcham Lavender' a term almost as famous as 'Scotch Whisky' or 'Ceylon Tea'. But the industry fell into decline in the Thirties, crippled partly by the ravages of *Phoma Lavandula* or shab, a disease which is fatal to lavender, and partly by the demand for housing in Mitcham, situated as it is on the outskirts of London; gradually the fields gave way to urban development. Although there are still elderly people living in the Mitcham district who can remember the comforting smell of lavender on the air whenever the distillery was working, today nothing whatsoever survives as a reminder of a remarkable era.

Despite the unhappy end to the industry in Mitcham, Linn Chilvers was convinced that there was still a market for quality lavender products. In 1932 he went into partnership with an equally enterprising local landowner, Ginger Dusgate, who made available the fields, while he provided the plants and expertise. Initially the harvest of lavender, laboriously cut by hand, had to be transported to Long Melford in the adjoining county of Suffolk, to have the essential oil extracted. But almost overnight the fortunes of the business were transformed by the arrival from Leicester of a chemist named Avery who possessed the secret recipe for a lavender water that had been made for King George IV some 130 years earlier. He offered to go into business with Linn Chilvers and supervise the making of the essence.

The successful sales of his perfume – which was personally bottled by Linn's two sisters Violet and Ivy using hand-held pipettes and bearing labels they stuck on – plus the introduction later of other lines including lavender bunches and talcum powder, built up the reputation of Norfolk Lavender. Soon they needed more land and their own distillery. With an ever-increasing number of customers, including Queen Mary, the grandmother of the present Queen, who came to Heacham to watch the harvest being brought in, Linn Chilvers knew his dream had been realised. When the chemist Avery died, his recipe was purchased by Norfolk Lavender and remains one of their staples to this day.

Mechanisation has entered into many aspects of lavender-farming since the Thirties. The harvesting, which takes about five or six weeks in July and August – the starting date dependent upon the amount of sunshine and rain on the crop during the preceding months – was formerly done by a team of about 40 people using the traditional sickle-shaped knives. As it is vital that the lavender is gathered when the bloom is at its best, long, exhausting hours were required of those in the harvesting teams. 'It was back-breaking work,' a former member, Peggy Emmerson, recalled, 'and we used to have to wear big straw hats and trousers because of the bees buzzing around us all the time. They loved the lavender. Everyone had to be careful that there wasn't a bee in the bush you were cutting – and make sure one didn't get in your clothes, either!'

It was not until 1964 that hand-picking was replaced by a rudimentary mechanical harvester; and not until 1970 that a purpose-built lavender-cutter was designed and made by a local agricultural engineering firm. According to Henry Head, this machine can cut four acres of lavender a day, which is almost exactly the same time it used to take a team of forty people. Henry was a great believer in the stamina-building power of lavender. 'I arrive at the office at 7.30 a.m. and don't leave before 6.30 p.m.' he told me. 'I'm sure it's all due to the lavender.'

To extract the essential oil from the lavender, in 1936 the company bought three French copper stills. Although stainless steel has replaced copper in all new stills, experts maintain that lavender distilled in copper produces a noticeably different oil; this is why Norfolk Lavender have continued to use the traditional method. The extraction process, carried out amidst the heady aroma of lavender, is one of the most enjoyable experiences to be had at Caley Mill.

On arriving fresh from the fields, the lavender, still complete with flowers and stalks, is carefully forked for any lurking bees before being tipped into the battery of large, cylindrical stills. These are slightly taller than a man and, as each one is filled up, a member of the four-strong team of loaders has to climb into the still to tread down the lavender. For years, a fine of ten shillings (50p) was levied on any man who injured a treader with his fork, the cash going to the aggrieved party.

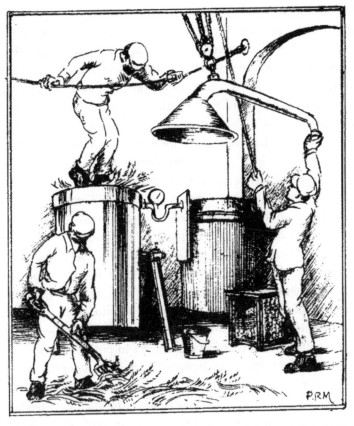

A lavender still being prepared for operation at Caley Mill (*Pip Miller*).

Once the still has been filled to the brim – it can take about a quarter of a ton (254 kilos) of lavender – the lid is securely fastened, and steam generated by an electric boiler is forced in under pressure. The value of retaining the stalks becomes evident during this part of the process because they help the steam to circulate and permeate the lavender. This causes the oil in the plant to vaporise and the mixture of oil vapour and steam passes by way of a projecting pipe at the top of the still to a second cylindrical container, the condenser, where it is cooled by circulating water and turns into a liquid once more. This is the pure essential oil of lavender – pale gold in colour – and it collects in the separator where it can be drawn off.

The entire distillation cycle, from forking in the lavender flowers to collecting the oil, takes about one hour, and the copper stills in Caley Mill can between them produce 1.5 to 3.5 litres (2½ to 6 pints) of essential oil during this period. The final act is to reopen the stills and the lavender, now blanched a light brown colour and of no further use, is unloaded in a cloud of aromatic steam which hangs tantalisingly in the air as the operation begins all over again. At the height of the season, the distillery works on a six-day rota for six weeks to distil 100 tons of lavender. Once the oil is collected, it is bottled and stored for about a year before being ready for sale or blending with other ingredients. 'We mature it like good wine,' said Henry Head, who estimates that it takes about five large bushes of lavender to produce one 10ml bottle (2 teaspoonfuls) of lavender oil.

The quality of the oil is dependent on the hours of sunshine the plant has received both before and during the harvest. And because each variety of lavender is quite different from the others and has its own distinctive fragrance and quality, this also comes into the equation where selection and growth at Norfolk Lavender are concerned. In the public gardens at Heacham, varieties can be seen in all their different shades from dark blue and purple to mauve, pink and white, with foliage varying from silvery grey to green or bright green. The purple varieties are said to have a stronger fragrance than the paler ones, and 'Imperial Gem' is said to be the most disease-free of all lavenders. During the distilling process the different varieties are kept quite separate from one another, and a series of hieroglyphics chalked on the side of each still indicates to the staff the precise spot on the rolling 100 acres where this batch originated.

In a storeroom adjoining the still, another 50 tons of lavender arrive load by load during the harvest – amounting to approximately one third of the crop – to be dried for use in pot-pourri, sachets and any of the company's many other products. In this 'drying-barn' the lavender is packed to half-fill sacks, laid in piles on the specially-built floor, and then left to dry at a temperature of 20°C (70°F) for about 36 hours. After that the flowers are ready for separating from the stalks and, finally, are sieved two or three times in a thresher. The stalks have no further use and are destroyed. People whose homes are in the vicinity of Caley Mill believe they must be among the very few living close to a manufacturing plant who actually love the smells issuing from it!

Because lavender produces its own insecticide, it is never sprayed with chemical pesticides at Heacham – and need not be in an ordinary garden either, according to the staff. Although it is a favourite with bees and butterflies, it is a repellent to greenfly and this pest is almost non-existent in the area. When visiting Caley Mill, gardening enthusiasts are often advised to plant lavender near their rose bushes as a guardian for their prize blooms against marauding greenfly. In fact, the company does not use sprays of any kind on its crops or test any of its products on animals: just two more reasons, it seems to me, why lavender is growing in popularity among all those who value the environment and its creatures.

Chapter 4
The Varieties of Lavender

The number of different species and cultivars of lavender has recently been quoted in otherwise authoritative works by horticulturalists and gardening experts as ranging from as few as two dozen to more than two hundred. Perhaps because the plant grows in so many different parts of the world, can hybridise easily, and some of the varieties look so alike to the inexperienced eye as to be almost identical, these discrepancies are to a degree understandable.

As Henry Head told me, it is actually very difficult to list the species of lavender because they have crossed with each other so much in the wild and, to make matters more complicated, their common names vary from country to country. But in England, he says, there are two main strains of straight-leaved lavenders most likely to be found in gardens:

1   *Lavandula latifolia* ('broad-leaved'). Tall, spike-headed shrubs with a pungent, camphoraceous scent and axial shoots growing from the main flower stems. Their leaves are broad greyish-green.
2   *Lavandula angustifolia* ('narrow-leaved'). These have short, stubby flower heads, each on an individual stalk. Their leaves are darker green, they have a sweeter fragrance and the oil is of a higher quality than in the *latifolias*.

There are reckoned to be literally hundreds of hybrids of *L. latifolia* and *L. angustifolia*, including a third group, *Lavandula X intermedia*, which are hybrids of both. These are large, branching plants with wide leaves, which were once much used in the Spanish oil industry. Not easy to find in nurseries in this country, the lavenders sold under that name are likely to be hybrids.

The simplest way to classify a lavender plant is probably by the axial shoots. Those which have them are strains of *latifolia* and those without are *angustifolia*.

Of all the cultivated lavenders, 'Hidcote' is perhaps the most popular with the general public, and a favourite of Alan Titchmarsh, a former presenter of the BBC's '*Gardeners' World*'. A variety of *angustifolia*, it is compact, often grown as a low hedge, and has violet-blue flowers with silver-grey leaves. It is ideal for use in flower arrangements and also in the making of lavender bags.

In contrast, there are several pink and white lavenders which are now available, including 'Loddon Pink' which has striking grey-green leaves, and the similar, slightly taller pink variety, 'Jean Davis'. The whites include the X *intermedia* 'Alba' and a dwarf *angustifolia* 'Nana Alba', with silver-grey foliage, which grows to a maximum of 38cm (15ins).

One of the most surprising facts I discovered about lavender is that such familiar names as 'French Lavender', 'Dutch Lavender', 'Italian Lavender' and, of course, 'English Lavender', which are quoted all over the world, are factually *incorrect*. There are actually *no* such botanical varieties – they are just lavenders that happen to be grown in those particular countries.

I am sorry to be the bearer of such disillusioning news, but Henry Head assures me that 'English Lavender' *only* means lavender grown in England, it is *not* a variety. The term 'French Lavender' is usually applied to *L. stoechas* and sometimes, confusingly, to Santolina chamaecyparissus, or cotton lavender, which belongs to a completely different botanical family.

It is because of the confusion that has arisen over the different lavenders that several national collections of lavender have been set up to bring together as many varieties as possible and cultivate them for reference and in the hope of some day compiling a definitive list. The collection at Heacham was the first of these, and all have been established under the auspices of the National Council for the Conservation of Plants and Gardens.

Finally, because I think it is important for gardeners to know whether any lavender plant they might buy at a nursery or garden centre is hardy and can cope with typical British conditions, or more tender and requires watching in the winter (perhaps even protecting from the elements), I have included the following list of commonly recognised lavenders and the categories into which they fall. It has been compiled with the assistance of Norfolk Lavender to whom I offer my grateful thanks.

Hardy Lavenders
L. angustifolia varieties

'Beechwood Blue'. Small compact bush, grey-green foliage, deep purple flowers (30–60 cm/12–24 ins).

'Folgate'. Compact shrub, narrow grey-green leaves, lavender-blue flowers (60 cm/24 ins).

'Folgate Blue'. Low, bushy shrub, thin green leaves, pale blue flowers (60 cm/24 ins).

'Heacham Blue'. Compact form, dark green leaves, dark blue to lavender shade flowers (60 cm/24 ins).

'Hidcote'. Small silvery bush, short, dark violet flowers (60–75 cm/24–30 ins).

'Imperial Gem'. Small shrub similar to 'Heacham Blue', dark green leaves, very deep purple flowers (60 cm/24 ins).

'Jean Davis'. Compact shrub, fresh green leaves, tiny pale pink flowers (60 cm/24 ins).

'Large White Flowered'. Long-stemmed variety with dark green leaves, striking white flowers (75 cm/30 ins).

'Loddon Blue'. Compact shrub, narrow greyish leaves, light blue flowers (60 cm/24 ins).

'Loddon Pink'. Compact form, narrow grey-green leaves, palest pink flowers (60 cm/24 ins).

'Munstead'. Dwarf form, narrow grey-green foliage, blue-purple flowers – bluer than most varieties (45–60 cm/18–24 ins).

'Nana Alba'. Compact mound, silvery-green leaves, white flowers (30-38 cm/12–15 ins).

'Nana Atropurpurea'. Similar to 'Hidcote', but an older form.

'Princess Blue'. Long-stemmed variety, dark green leaves, light blue flowers (70 cm/28 ins).

'Rosea'. Compact form, narrow grey-green leaves, lavender-pink flowers (75 cm/30 ins).

'Royal Purple'. Small bush, narrow green leaves, vivid purple flowers (60-75 cm/24–30 ins).

'Twickel Purple'. Narrow oblong leaves, purple flowers (60 cm–1 m/ 24–39 ins).

'Vera.' Large silvery-white bush, lavender-blue flowers (90 cm/36 ins).

L. X intermedia varieties

'Alba'. Robust, tall variety, grey-green leaves, white flowers (90 cm/ 36 ins).

'Dutch'. Medium shrub, straight-leaved hybrid, purple-blue flowers (75 cm/30 ins). Both 'Dutch' and 'Old English' (see below) are often confused with each other and sold as *L. spica*, a name which should not now be used.

'Grappenhall'. Broad grey-green leaves, lavender-blue flowers on long spikes (1 m/39 ins).

'Grey Hedge'. Spreading bushy shrub, grey-green leaves, greyish-white flowers (45 cm/18 ins).

'Grosso'. Tall variety, straight grey-green leaves, laden with blue-purple flowers (90 cm/36 ins).

'Hidcote Giant'. Similar to 'Grappenhall', but with darker flowers.

'Old English'. Medium shrub, larger than 'Dutch' (see above), with straight green leaves and purple flowers.

'Seal'. Rounded shrub, broad silvery-grey leaves, pale purple flowers.

L. latifolia variety

'Spikenard'. Compact bush, largish silvery-grey leaves and fat, dark purple flowers. A very fragrant lavender now grown mainly for use in perfume (60 cm/24 ins).

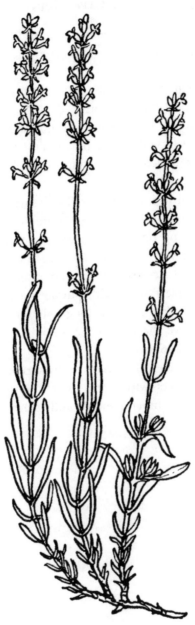

A typical variety of the lavender plant, *Lavandula angustifolia* 'Vera' (*British Pharmacopoeia*, 1924).

Tender Lavenders

L. allardii. Largest of the lavenders, scalloped dark green leaves, tightly packed deep-purple flowers curved and tapered at the top (1 m/39 ins).

L. canariensis. Medium-sized bushy shrub, ferny green leaves, bright blue flowers (75-90 cm/30–36 ins).

L. dentata. Spreading, bushy shrub, scalloped dark green leaves, purple-blue flowers with purple bracts (1 m/39 ins).

L. lanata. Small rounded shrub, white woolly leaves, dark purple flowers (75–90 cm/30–36 ins).

L. multifida. Similar to *L. canariensis.* Bushy shrub with ferny green leaves and blue-purple flowers (75–90 cm/30–36 ins).

L. pinnata. Spreading bushy shrub, grey-green leaves covered in white hairs, blue-purple flowers (60 cm/24 ins).

L. stoechas (French Lavender). Dwarf, very aromatic shrub, narrow leaves, dark purple flowers with purple bracts (45 cm/18 ins). Subspecies *L.s. pedunculata* has longer flower stalks holding the flowers well above the foliage. Commonly known as 'Spanish Lavender' (35 cm/26 ins).

L. viridis. (Green Lavender). Upright bushy shrub, pale green leaves, small white flowers with green bracts. Originally from the Pyrenees, it is temperamental and slow-growing (60–75 cm/24–30 ins).

PART 2
Using Lavender

Chapter 5
How Does Your Lavender Grow?

Roald Dahl, author of several of the most famous of modern children's books, including *Charlie and the Chocolate Factory* and *James and the Giant Peach*, was just one of countless gardeners who hold lavender in high regard. In the years prior to his death in 1990, he grew a combination of four varieties of the plant down both sides of a path in his garden at Great Missenden in Buckinghamshire. Often in the mornings, as he strode from the house to the small hut at the end of the garden where he wrote all his books, he would pause to admire the array of purple flowers. Occasionally he showed off the borders to favoured friends and visitors, and it is not really surprising that the herb even found its way into some of his stories.

Gertrude Jekyll, the doyenne of gardening authorities, was if anything an even greater admirer of the plant. In 1900 she wrote in her book *Home and Garden*, 'A whole garden could be planted with lavender alone to represent hard-wooded, shrubby growth.' In her earlier volume, *Wood and Garden* (1899), she had enthused: 'To reap the fragrant harvest of lavender is one of the joys of the flower year. If it is to be kept and dried, it should be cut when as yet only a few of the purple blooms are out on the spike; if left too late, the flower shakes off the stalk too readily.'

One of the best known of all lavenders, the dwarf variety 'Munstead', was named after Gertrude Jekyll's cottage home. There, throughout her life, she liked to edge her paths with the compact, low-growing variety, resplendent with its deep blue flowers. Those who knew her said that the plant was a lilting tribute to her own sparkling blue eyes.

What both Gertrude Jekyll and Roald Dahl appreciated was that although lavender is hardy, long-lived and resilient, able to thrive on stony ground and requiring little fuss to be made of it, it *does* need a certain amount of care and attention to get the best results. The points to bear in mind especially are these:

- Lavender grows best in an alkaline soil that is well drained.

- Lavender requires plenty of fresh air and sunshine. Alan Titchmarsh says, 'It needs a sun-drenched spot to prevent it becoming leggy, and to release its essential oils.'

- Lavender will not grow well in shade where it is prone to fungal diseases.

- Lavender can be grown from seed and cuttings.

- Lavender bushes can be planted singly or as a hedge.

In many parts of the British Isles the plant has come to be regarded as the archetypal symbol of the country garden, especially on hot summer days when it is alive with industrious honey bees and beautiful butterflies, and full of that delicious fragrance that can bring a sense of peace and harmony to the whole vicinity. Planted on its own, the lavender's domed top is more evident than in a hedge, but either way it offers as much as three months of splendid floral display and a grey-green foliage that is eye-catching all year long.

Sites

When selecting a site in your garden to grow lavender, ensure, first, that it is in sunlight all day long and does not collect water; if the soil is at all acid, mulch it well with lime before planting. Where the ground is very heavy, cut a trench for the plant and line this with shingle to facilitate drainage. Do try to find the nearest to an ideal position for lavender, or the spikes will be weak, overlong and fewer in number. An unsuitable location can also mean that the general appearance of your lavender will be poor and the aroma far less pleasing. The best time of year for planting is between September and March and, where you intend the herb to form an 'evergrey' hedge, set the young plants about 30 cm (12 ins) apart.

The final choice of location is, of course, your decision, but here are a few points to bear in mind when picking which variety to plant. The two most familiar species, *L. angustifolia* and *L. latifolia*, grow best on terraced sites, if well spaced rather than crowded together; while *L. dentata* and *L. stoechas* are renowned for swiftly covering sloping sites. They will also self-sow.

Germination

Although lavender can be grown from seed, it is as well to be aware that germination is often slow. Seeds are, of course, available from most garden centres and seedsmen, but they can be taken from the flowers of the plant when they are being pruned. Because lavender hybridises easily, plants grown from seed are not always true to type, producing interesting if occasionally unexpected results that may be quite different from the parent.

Propagation

Growing lavender from cuttings should be carried out in March or October for best results, although any time during spring or autumn is permissible with such a hardy plant. For your cuttings select ripe young shoots between 10 and 20 cm (4 and 8 ins) in length, which are springing from the sides of older branches and as yet have no flower buds. Pull them off gently downwards so that some of the old wood comes away with each cutting to form a 'heel'.

These new cuttings will root well in clay pots of light, sandy compost which can be kept in a cold frame or greenhouse, or even indoors if you intend to grow one of the tender varieties. But thanks to modern rooting hormone compounds they can be grown just as successfully in the open. To facilitate this, dig a trench, about 10 cm (4 ins) deep and 20 cm (8 ins) wide, in a bed that is not too exposed to the elements, and half-fill it with equal parts of sand and garden soil mixed well together. After dipping the cut stems in the hormone compound, insert them firmly into the trench to about half their length, each about 10 cm (4 ins) apart. Moisten the cuttings well and cover with clear polythene, supported on sticks, which should be staked down against the wind, or use a tunnel cloche. Remove this about twice a week in the evenings to moisten the cuttings. The polythene can be left off during the day when the cuttings show signs of growth, and after about six weeks may be dispensed with altogether. Cuttings planted in the spring are generally said to root the quickest.

After six months, replant those cuttings which have rooted successfully in ordinary garden soil, again spacing them about 10 cm (4 ins) apart, and allow about 20 cm (8 ins) between the rows in order to give the plant room to grow plump and be ready for putting out the following autumn. When a year old, the new plants should be cut back after they have flowered to encourage bushy growth. After two years, the young lavenders are ready for a permanent place in your chosen location.

A simpler although less predictable method of propagation is to bend over some of the lower stems of a mature bush and mound soil over them, leaving the tip visible. This method, known as 'layering', takes about six months to produce results, and meanwhile it may be necessary to ensure that the stem is kept under the earth with a brick on top of the soil. Once the stem has rooted (the evidence of this will be a healthy green shoot), it can be cut off from the main stem and transplanted elsewhere. One drawback of 'layering' is that the plants are usually not as well-shaped as those grown from cuttings.

Although, as I mentioned, lavender can thrive in poor soils, a little compost will help to encourage growth. On heavy clay, for example, compost or manure is recommended; while on sandy soil the plant will benefit from a mixture of coarse bonemeal and lime. For thin soil over chalk, bonemeal alone will suffice. At Norfolk Lavender they warned me that although a high potash feed promotes flowering, a soil that is too rich in nitrogen may result in limp plants with too much leafy growth.

Pruning

After its annual flowering, an established lavender hedge will benefit from pruning to keep it from growing untidy and too 'woody'. The dead flower spikes along with up to 8 cm (3 ins) of stem growth should be clipped off to even the top and sides. Dead branches should be removed entirely, cutting back to clean, living wood. Some gardeners believe that a good tonic for ageing lavender is to scatter dried farmyard manure sludge (about 250g or 8 oz per square metre or yard) around the plants and then water this into the ground.

Lavender hedges that have been neglected but are still strong can be cut to shape in October, using a saw on the thick branches and taking them to about 8 cm (3 ins) from the ground. This should enable the plants to grow afresh from the base. Some experts prefer this cutting to be done in spring after the danger of frost has decreased, but not later than March or there is a danger that the flowering will suffer. If the 'sludge tonic' is used in conjunction with this exercise, it will help produce new shoots on the bare branches and encourage general all-round new life for the lavender plants.

A tip about the branches you have pruned. Don't just throw them away on the compost heap, because the oil content will slow down the decomposing process. It's better to burn them on the household fire because the fragrance is wonderful and a perfect reminder, as you toast your toes, of long, hot summer days! I am also told that the scented stems were once burnt by country people like joss sticks.

In the past, many experts were inclined to the view that lavender bushes should only be kept for three flowering years and then pulled up and destroyed. Today there are those who maintain that the plants should be pulled up and replaced every six years. In my estimation, it is the way the plant is cared for that should determine its life span – a view that is certainly shared at Norfolk Lavender where they strongly discourage wholesale removal of bushes that may have years of life left in them.

Pests

For centuries gardeners have believed that the strong smell of lavender keeps pests away, and this has earned it a favourable reputation among many of those who grow vegetables and fruit. Certainly, planting it near such crops does seem to keep away the worst pests, especially those that prey on succulent garden plants.

Only one pest is immune to the aromatic smell of lavender: the green capsid bug (still known in some country districts as the frog-hopper) which produces the white deposits aptly named cuckoo spit. Although this may *look* unpleasant, it is actually quite harmless to the lavender.

Disease

Disease can attack the lavender bush in several ways. Frost, for instance, may injure shoots and cause them to die back. Infected tissues may be attacked by grey mould which shows as a grey, velvety growth on dead shoots. This fungus may also attack the flowers during a wet season, causing them to wilt or turn brown prematurely. According to some authorities lavender can be harmed by honey fungus and leaf spot may appear as small spots on the leaves, although neither has been very noticeable in recent years.

The only killer disease is shab (*Phoma Lavandula*) which appears as tiny black spots on the stems. These spores attack the flower stalks, causing them to wind into corkscrew shapes and turn brown. After this, parts of the bush die and urgent attention is required because there is no cure for shab. The shrub must be removed and destroyed before the disease spreads to any other lavender bushes. According to the experts, most of the modern hybrids have become resistant to shab, although two types, 'Munstead' and 'Loddon Pink', are still susceptible. An old countryman also told me that dogs allowed to urinate on lavender bushes on a regular basis can kill them.

Harvesting and drying

Lavender has the unique distinction of being the only herb that can be used fresh from the garden and laid on clothes or linen without fear of marking. It will also dry quite naturally in most of the living-rooms of the house; the stems remain strong, and neither colour nor fragrance will disappear for some time. And when they do, there is a fading elegance quite unlike any other dried plant. There are, in my estimation, very few better flowers for dried arrangements than lavender: it is much less brittle than others, and few decorative plants have such a scent all their own.

However, those lavender flowers which you wish to dry should be picked when the blooms are showing colour but before they are fully opened – ideally, on a summer morning after the dew has evaporated and the buds are beginning to open. Use scissors to cut the whole flower stalks, tie them in bunches with a piece of ribbon, tape or strong elastic band, and then hang in a dry, airy place out of direct sunlight, as this will cause the colour to fade. Because the stems will shrink while drying, keep an eye out for any that drop out of their binding; you can tell when the process is complete because the flowers will crackle to the touch. They are now ready for stripping and using in lavender bags, sachets and so on.

Another method that has been recommended to me is laying the stems no more than three deep in shallow cardboard boxes which are then stacked in a dry place, one upon the other and in alternate directions to allow the air to circulate. This drying process should take about a fortnight if the boxes are in a shady spot. Do not put them in the sun as this wastes the scent. The same goes for an airing cupboard, *unless* you are happy for it to smell very strongly of lavender.

If you are planning to use lavender in summer cooking, you may prefer to dry the flowers in the oven. To do this, place the required number of spikes on a piece of brown paper (to absorb the moisture) and leave in the oven for about one hour at 50°C (120°F). They will then be ready for you to crumble directly onto the other ingredients for your recipe. (The same result can be achieved by putting the lavender on its brown paper into the microwave and leaving it for about a minute at high.)

Lavender leaves can, of course, be picked at any time, and an afternoon stroll around the garden in the depths of winter can be enlivened by plucking and squeezing them as you check that all is well with the plants for spring.

Gertrude Jekyll has written with feeling of this whole business of lavender harvesting. 'The lavender crop is carefully watched and harvested at the moment of its best early maturity,' she declared in *Home and Garden.* 'This is when a good number of the lower flowers in the spike are open, but none of those in the top. We arrange to have the two hedges that are in bearing in such positions that one is in a rather warmer aspect than the other, so that the whole crop does not come ripe at the same time.'

Locations

The most popular way of growing lavender is undoubtedly as an edging for paths – in the style of Roald Dahl – or at the front of beds or borders. It is also a staple in most herb gardens and increasingly popular in knot gardens, too. There is even a place for it in tiny suburban gardens or the very smallest city balcony or windowbox.

Geoff Hamilton, the popular TV gardener and writer who died in 1996, firmly believed that the cottage garden style, which has endured in one form or another in England since the Middle Ages, could be adapted for gardens anywhere by utilising the right plants. He maintained that lavender was among the most important of these – typifying the past while at the same time offering by-products for the present and future.

Because the paths in so many modern gardens are made of gravel with concrete or timber edging, or else with bricks or paving slabs, he felt that the ideal way of disguising the formal edges was with a low-growing plant like lavender. He thought, and I agree with him, that the best variety for the job was the dwarf shrub, 'Munstead', which so attractively softens a path's rigid lines.

To obtain the best effect in borders it is important to select the right plants. Roses and lavender are considered ideal for the front, while the back should be left to shrubs and the taller herbaceous plants. Talking about lavender in this context, Geoff Hamilton said in one of his programmes, 'There are now many different varieties, like the white 'Alba' and the vigorous lavender-blue 'Grappenhall'. If you want to mix colours, there are also several pink varieties such as 'Loddon Pink' and 'Hidcote Pink'. But none, in my view, is as satisfactory as the traditional lavender-blue varieties.'

Some gardeners like to plant lavender near a seat or summer-house so that anyone sitting there can enjoy the sight and smell of the plants. But rather than having just lavender in such a location, why not group it with several other plants, such as scented stocks, garden pinks, hyssop, thyme and perhaps even a bush or two of old roses? Alan Titchmarsh says, 'Lavender is the perfect companion for roses, its pastel colouring being a perfect foil for the brighter rose flowers, releasing its fragrance when you brush past it.'

Herb and Knot Gardens

If you have space for a herb garden, surrounded by either a wall or a thick hedge, lavender is best located where the sun shines longest and the ground is driest. The plant has no objection to sharing a bed with several other popular herbs, including rosemary, caraway and chervil.

Lavender is equally at home in a knot garden – a kind of miniature world of intertwined low hedges which first became popular in the fifteenth century. Following a decline of interest for about two hundred years, knot gardens are now becoming increasingly popular again among imaginative gardeners. The early patterns were very complicated, with the hedging crisscrossing the rectangular shape both above and below itself to give the appearance of knotted threads. The spaces in between were filled with coloured gravel or flowering plants. Knot gardens were almost always built close to a house, so that they could be viewed with equal pleasure from an upper window or a ground floor room.

The formality of the design has meant that, of all period gardening devices, the knot is ideally suited to a modern garden *regardless* of its size. In fact, few other designs make such effective use of a small space. And by including flower colours that change through the season to delight the eye, and a selection of aromatic plants which are pleasant to touch and smell, a knot garden can provide continual interest and enjoyment. The sketch shown here, of a typical sixteenth-century knot garden, could be a starting-point for your own design.

It is obviously important to select plants for the knot carefully, taking into consideration such factors as their hardiness, speed of growth, amount of maintenance and, particularly, the all-year-round interest they provide. Not surprisingly, I think, lavender was one of the earliest favourites – along with box, yew and rosemary – and it has retained its popularity. The dwarf lavender 'Hidcote' comes highly recommended. I have seen a knot garden as tiny as 1.5 metres (5 feet) square, consisting of dwarf box, golden foliage thuja and three different varieties of lavender, so no matter how tiny your plot may be, there could still be room for one on your property.

Balconies and ledges

Finally, we come to the use of lavender in a flat or apartment which has only a small balcony or window ledge. The ideal solution for a balcony is a tub filled with a selection of different varieties of lavender, their number really dependent on the size of the container. A good selection would be a grouping of L. *stoechas* with a dwarf L. *angustifolia* and some heliotrope or 'Cherry Pie' as it is commonly known, due to its scent. The combination is an aromatic delight! The plants should be bedded in a well-drained soil or compost, and put in the sunniest spot for the summer months. Some experts suggest that, if the balcony is very exposed, the tub will have to come indoors during the winter – when you might like to consider changing the 'Cherry Pie' for one or other of the herbs that combine well with lavender and also suit your taste in fragrances.

In the case of a really small flat you may well have to settle for a single lavender plant in a clay pot. Choose whichever variety you like

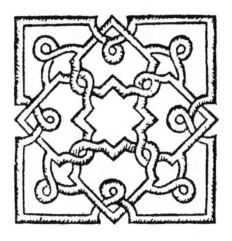

Outline plan for a knot garden from a sixteenth-century gardening manual (*The Gardener's Labyrinth*, 1560).

best, and don't feel you *have* to put the plant on the window sill – a place beside the door where people come and go can be even more suitable, because here everyone who brushes by the lavender will release a little of that unforgettable aroma and bring some sunshine into their lives – and yours!

Chapter 6
Lavender at Home and Work

The many different qualities and versatility of lavender have traditionally given it a special place in the home. Back in the seventeenth century, for instance, Izaak Walton, who worked as a linen-draper before writing his masterpiece, *The Compleat Angler* (1653), declared with all the enthusiasm of personal experience and no little expectation, 'Let's go to that house, for the linen looks white and smells of lavender, and I long to lie in a pair of sheets that smell so.' The Victorian novelist Elizabeth Gaskell, who was noted almost as much for her great beauty and sweetness of disposition as for her best-selling romantic novels, was the daughter of a boarding-house keeper who prided himself on his spotless establishment. In her novel *Cranford* (1853) she referred wistfully to the 'little bunches of lavender flowers sent to strew the drawers of some town dweller, or to burn in the room of some invalid.'

Although the thought of burning lavender in a sickroom, to 'disinfect and sweeten the air', may seem a little odd to some readers, there are quite a number of uses to which lavender can be put in the home, which have been tried and tested over the years and are now finding acceptance all over the world. In 1953, for example, we find Colette, the great French novelist and recorder of sensual experiences, taking pains to conjure up the versatility of the plant in her book *Bella Vista*, when she writes of 'the smell of lavender, dried bunches of which hung on the bedrail and in the cupboard and made life pleasant for those who lived in the house.'

To its many admirers, the scent of lavender comes closest to encapsulating the caring and comforting qualities of home. Its unique fresh and spicy scent carries echoes of the cleanliness and purity that everyone seeks in their daily lives, both within the four walls of home and, to a different degree, at work.

Quite a number of family doctors, along with herbalists and alternative therapists, have accepted that lavender has special qualities that can be utilised in a practical way to enhance people's lives as well as their environment. Whether this amounts to nothing more than an arrangement of fresh flowers in a vase or a generous bunch of the herb to perfume and freshen the air, or to a complex blend of essential oils chosen to benefit health and well-being, lavender has an important role to play. The suggestions below can be followed as they are, or adapted and varied to suit your own requirements.

Lavender Oil

At Home

A fresh aroma around the home is surely one of the most basic of all requirements, making it a pleasant place to live in and return to after a hard day at work. One of the most effective and pleasing ways of doing this is to use an essential oil burner or vaporiser. These attractive little pieces of equipment, which are generally chimney-shaped and made from clay (occasionally glass, porcelain or marble) have on top a small bowl for the oil and water. There is also a hole on one side to allow the air to circulate around the nightlight which heats the bowl and causes the oil to vaporise, so spreading its fragrance into the air.

Alternatively, there are two more sophisticated kinds of vaporiser. The electric fragrancer uses undiluted essential oil dripped onto a filter surface (usually made of ceramic) which is kept at a constant warm temperature to release the vapour. The steam diffuser is worked by a cold-air pump which blows tiny droplets of the neat oil into the air.

Lavender oil is ideal for use as a general air freshener and I would recommend a formula of four teaspoons of water to eight drops of lavender. When heated in the bowl, this will give you at least two hours of delightful fragrance. But a word of caution. Do ensure that the bowl is not too near the heat or it could burn, and keep an eye on the water level. Replenish the lavender oil and water as necessary. In the case of the electric vaporiser, four drops of lavender oil at a time will perfume the average room quite satisfactorily.

All these diffusers release the lavender oil molecules into the air to create a pleasant aroma, but are equally good at killing off airborne bacteria and combating the unpleasant odours of cigarettes, animals and after-cooking smells.

If you are spending the day at home, then vaporising a blend of lavender and two other essential oils can put you in the right frame of mind, regardless of whether you just want a little peace and quiet or are intending to be more active with chores and other tasks. If rest is your main requirement, burn a mixture of four drops each of lavender and sandalwood with two of geranium, but if you want to get into a party mood you need a combination of four drops each of orange and eucalyptus oil added to two of lavender.

Another method of filling a room with the fragrance of lavender – especially in the winter – was told me by a friend who recommended hanging a bunch of dried lavender which had been sprinkled with a few drops of lavender oil on a radiator. The warmth of the radiator then gradually releases the fragrance into the room. I have heard that in Canada they do much the same thing with pine cones strung together and impregnated with lavender oil. As the heat penetrates these 'fragrant cones' it causes them gradually to open and release the mingled pine and lavender aromas into the atmosphere.

Adding a few drops of lavender oil to the wax of a burning candle can also freshen a room. Obviously you require a fairly big candle which produces plenty of wax, and **you must take care when adding the lavender oil because it is flammable.** First light the candle and allow some melted wax to accumulate before extinguishing the flame. Next, add two to three drops of lavender oil around the wick and relight the candle. Watch to see that the wick is kept short so that it does not produce too large a flame and vaporise the oil too quickly. And **never** add the oil while the candle is alight, for if you do it will flare up in a puff of black smoke! The result of taking care is a candle-lit evening which smells delicious!

Which rooms you decide to scent in this way will obviously be a matter of personal taste. As a general rule, lavender is said to be most suitable for use in the living-room, sitting-room, bathroom, lavatory and bedroom. In all of these the oil may be burned on its own, in a blend with other compatible oils, or even with proprietary products.

In any room, it is important always to bear in mind the kind of mood you want to create, and this is especially true of the living-room and sitting-room. Here relaxation is the key word and this is best created by putting the vaporiser to work for an hour or two *before* you settle down for the evening. Because these rooms generally bring together the largest number of people for the longest period of time, I would recommend a blend of oils, the best in my experience being lavender, petitgrain and clary sage.

In the bathroom it is vital to ensure that everything is always kept clean and fragrant. When mopping up the bath or cleaning the floor, add two or three drops of lavender to your hot water to act as a cleaner *and* disinfectant. Rinse the same amount around the wash basin to ensure that it is germ-free, too. If you use one of the vaporisers before a bath and fancy a blend of oils rather than lavender on its own, then a mixture of lavender, geranium and petitgrain in the condenser will create a pleasing effect. Lavender oil can also, of course, be added to the bathwater to ease a number of complaints, and these are discussed in Chapter Seven.

A friend who has only a shower in her flat has discovered a novel method of making the most of lavender oil whenever she showers. She puts a flannel over the drain and then sprinkles ten drops of oil over the shower base. The flannel prevents the hot water rushing away and as the steam rises it swirls the lavender fragrance all around her. The combination of warm water on the skin and breathing in the lavender is, she says, just heavenly!

Hygiene is even more important in the lavatory. Here you can choose between a pot-pourri, lavender bag or vaporiser to provide general freshness. Sprinkling a few drops of the essential oil into the lavatory bowl is also recommended. A most suitable blend of oils for use in a burner in the smallest room is lavender, pine and lemon. Even the aroma of tea tree – which is very strong – works here when blended with the other three. It also aids in the general disinfectant process.

When it comes to the bedrooms, a careful distinction must be made between those in which adults sleep and those used by children. For men and women, a blend of lavender, camomile and clary sage is good in the vaporiser, but the amounts of oil should be halved when used in any room where youngsters sleep. It is safer to use an electric diffuser for children rather than the nightlight burner. Lavender can be put to work in various other ways to scent the bedroom as well as to protect clothes, linen and so on, and details of these uses are given later in this chapter.

Moving house can be made decidedly more fragrant with the assistance of lavender. As soon as you take over the property – new or old – set your vaporiser to work and move it from one room to the next until each has been treated. Lavender oil on its own or a blend of equal amounts of lavender and juniper are recommended for this process, and it is the quickest way I know to re-create a familiar and comforting atmosphere and make you feel 'at home' in your new surroundings.

The Workplace

The aroma you create at home for your own convenience is one thing; at work, unless you have an office to yourself, the situation may be quite different. Lavender may not be to everyone's liking, and you should certainly seek the approval of colleagues before introducing a perfume to the place that may well put you in a great mood for work but simply irritates them. Research has shown that the fragrances that are acceptable to the widest range of people are those from either the green or the citrus families – that is essences like pine, cypress, juniper, lemon, lime, orange, grapefruit and so on. The reason for this is that the green scents engender a welcome feeling of the great outdoors for people cooped up inside, while the citrus essences are uplifting.

If you do have the opportunity to use a vaporiser at work, the electric diffuser is obviously less of a fire risk than the candle burner. Apart from making the office fragrant, these little gadgets make excellent fumigators and help prevent the spread of bacteria in workplaces which, these days, are often crowded and stuffy. They are probably at their most invaluable in the winter when, as we all know, every other person seems to have a cold.

My ideal blend for the office vaporiser would be a mixture of lavender, rosemary and grapefruit oils in which no one scent overpowers the other and the fragrance is effective while at the same time being unobtrusive. Try it and see!

Lavender fresh or dried

Bunches

Lavender bunches are probably the most familiar and certainly the simplest by-product of the plant for use in the home. Because they grow anything up to 90cm (3 ft) long, stems of lavender can be cut to any length and are suitable for utilising in small sprigs or large bundles. The former look good hanging from bedheads, curtain rails or picture frames, while the latter can be draped on doors, around window frames or from the ceiling. I would recommend that when tying up your lavender bunch you use a complementary material such as old-fashioned rayon ribbons, raffia or embroidery threads to enhance the effect. Another attractive use is to cut a substantial bundle of straight, firm stems all the same length – ideally from one of the dwarf varieties with the stalks about twice the length of the flowered part – fasten the bundle in the middle with a decorative thread and stand upright like a miniature corn stook. This particular lavender creation can make a most attractive table or sideboard display. When dried out, the lavender flowers need not be thrown away but can be used in a number of the following ways:

Scent Bags

I could not resist including the following instructions for the making of a 'lavender scent bag' which I came across some years ago in an old Victorian book entitled *Grandmama's Secrets*, published in 1856, which was intended to be put in a young lady's trousseau before her wedding in order to help her in married life. The language is so quaint that I suspect it was reprinted from an earlier source:

Take of lavender flowers, free from stalk, half a pound; dried thyme and mint, of each half an ounce; ground cloves and caraways, of each a quarter of an ounce; common salt, dried, one ounce; mix the whole well together, and put the product into silk or cambric bags. In this way it will perfume the drawers and linen very nicely.

Sachets

The plain lavender bag is by far the most popular scented item for putting in drawers and amongst clothes. Experience has taught me that for the most efficient sachets, the lavender should be picked just before it is in full bloom and early in the morning, when the dew has gone but the sun's rays have not had time to evaporate the scent from the blossoms. The more mature the plant, the better its fragrance. There are lots of ways of drying lavender, some of which I have already described in the previous chapter, but just make sure you put the cuttings in a warmish, airy place and never in direct sunlight because the sunshine can draw out much of the precious aroma. Some experts recommend covering the cuttings with brown paper which will prevent the flowers from fading. Once the lavender is dry, rub the tiny flowers off the stalks. These should be placed either in your ready-made sachets or in an airtight jar to retain the scent. Lavender-coloured muslin or silk organdie bags, their tops drawn in with a bow or ribbon, have proved enduringly popular, but never be afraid of using your imagination where colours and materials are concerned. Just remember that gauzy fabrics are the best. Over the years I have seen any number of sachets, from tiny lace-edged bags to larger heart-shaped creations – many made from traditional sprigged muslin in pastel shades, or from plain organza in hues of pink, mauve and blue. Some of the most attractive have also been embroidered in silk. You can be sure with all of these that the fragrance of the lavender will last for many months, and in any event can always be replenished the following year after the harvest.

Drawer-liners

Lavender-scented drawer-liners are an alternative to sachets and are easy to make. First choose a suitable sheet of decorated paper (remnants of wall-paper are excellent) and cut it to the size of the drawer. Next cover the back with a thin layer of glue and sprinkle onto it a thick layer of dried lavender flowers. Press these down with your fingers and then leave the glue to dry. Shake off any flowers that have not stuck to the paper and then place *flower side down* into the drawer. The drawer is now ready for use – and it is a good idea each time you open it to rub your hands lightly over the sheet in order to release more of the delightful fragrance from the underside.

Posies

Lavender posies are a useful idea which apparently originated in France, where they are put among sheets in the linen cupboard. The lavender should again be cut just before the flowers open, but ensure that you have long stems and that the flowers are really fresh, for dried lavender is too brittle and you will be unable to mould the stems properly. Next divide the cuttings into bundles of 15 and tie them firmly just below the flowers. Bend an uneven number of the stalks over the flower-heads to form a 'cage' and thread a ribbon in and out of the stems from top to bottom to form a basketweave pattern. Secure each end of the ribbon with a bow and the posies are then ready for the cupboard.

Bottles

These are an English version of the posies, which have been made in country districts for many years. They are known in some parts of Southern England as lavender cones. Once again, ensure that the lavender you are going to use is fresh. You will require 30 heads and a piece of ribbon 3mm ($^1/_8$ in) wide and 106 cm (3ft 6in) long for each bottle. Tie the heads together just below the flowers with the ribbon. Now gently bend the stalks over the flowers and begin interweaving the ribbon through alternate stalks, continuing around the stalks until all the flowers are enclosed. Finally, twist the ribbon several times round the stalks to secure them, knot the ribbon and cut it. Secure with a needle and thread. What makes the lavender bottle particularly attractive is the fact that the dried stems have the appearance of fine wicker and this is enhanced by the colourful ribbon. Although ideal for the linen drawer, these bottles can easily be hung up in cupboards by a loop attached to the ribbon.

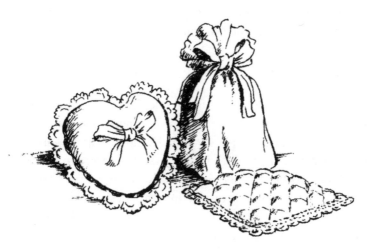

Lavender bags have been among the most popular items
utilising the herb for centuries. (*Pip Miller*).

Pot-pourri

In most households I have visited, the lavender pot-pourri consists of just that – a shallow bowl brimming with dried lavender. But with the addition of a fixative and some of the essential oil, a pot-pourri can be made to last a good deal longer. If you are going to try to create your own mixture of aromatic flowers, time and experiment are probably the best guidelines – although I would recommend the following ingredients as being well worth a trial. You will need a cup of dried lavender flowers; half a cup of dried marjoram leaves; a tablespoon each of orris root powder, dried thyme leaves and mint leaves; two teaspoons of ground coriander and a quarter of a teaspoon of ground cloves. This particular mixture also benefits from the addition of a few drops of lavender oil. First mix the flowers and leaves together. Next blend the orris powder (which helps to 'fix' the other ingredients), coriander and cloves in a separate bowl, stirring in the lavender oil. Lastly add this mixture to the dried material and place in your pot-pourri container which could be a china plate, earthenware crock or glass jar. **Never** use a plastic or aluminium container as these will undermine the fragrance. (Some experts suggest storing the mixture in a sealed jar in a cool, dark place for up to a month to 'cure' before putting it to use – but that is only if you can wait that long!)

Baskets

A lavender basket is one of the glories of summer flower arrangements – and one that will last a lot longer than many others. Indeed, I have heard people say that lavender is as important to summer decoration as holly is to Christmas. Some professional floral decorators use lavender in garlands, swags, wreaths and even ornamental trees, but the instructions for designs like these are rather too complex and time-consuming to be included in an introductory book such as this. The basket of lavender flowers is, however, quite a different matter. The easiest type to create needs no more than a floral foam block (or blocks) to line the bottom of a wickerwork basket, the older, more traditional types being preferable. Insert into the block as many stems of lavender as you can, cutting them all to the same length to emphasise the striking regularity of the plant. Some flower arrangers prefer to mix different types and colours of lavender in their baskets, while others sometimes combine different flower-heads and even traditional greenery as the fancy takes them. Fresh lavender flowers make a beautiful, scented display, and after they have dried can be turned to other uses, too.

Cushions

Elaborately decorated lavender cushions were being made as early as the fourteenth century: Charles VI of France was particularly fond of them and ordered dozens to be made for his apartments. The king's cushions were made of white satin with the dried lavender flowers mixed in amongst the stuffing to provide a fragrant aroma for the royal nostrils as he reclined upon them. Today, with most cushions being easy to open, it is perhaps more practical to insert the dried lavender into them in a small muslin bag. In this way it will be simpler to replace the lavender whenever necessary.

Pillows

Country lore has long claimed that lavender pillows are a great aid to sleep – they will drive away nightmares and guarantee you sweet dreams. Centuries before the advent of the mattress, many people slept on bedding consisting of straw in a linen sack and nothing could have been more natural than to mix in some sweet-smelling and soothing lavender with the straw. This tradition has survived with the pillow, and by stuffing fresh lavender flowers inside the filling it should remain fragrant for at least two years. I am told that some people occasionally augment the aroma in the pillow with a drop or two of lavender oil on the fabric. A lavender pillow is also said to be good for overcoming nausea and travel sickness.

Insect Repellents

Lavender is particularly good at keeping moths, silverfish and other insects away from clothes and linen, as well as driving out musty smells from storage spaces. Both sachets and bundles of dried flowers will help in this unceasing campaign. Trial and experience have shown that for sachets a mixture of two parts of lavender to four of tansy and southernwood (that is, field southernwood or artemisia), plus one of rosemary and a half-measure of powdered orris root to act as the fixative, makes up an effective repellent. Our forebears, who made herb bunches to hang over their beds or in cupboards, would use a bunch of lavender as the base and add two stems of southernwood, one of hyssop and several red roses. These bundles have to be made while the plants are still fresh and they should be tied together with a ribbon before hanging up. They will remain effective for months.

Scented Coat-hangers

A lavender-scented coat-hanger is another useful weapon in the war against insects, and it also freshens the environment at the same time. First, make a muslin bag the length of a wooden coat-hanger and fill it with the same mixture as for the sachet in the previous section. Now, after covering the hanger with a plain material, sew the muslin bag onto it and finally wrap over it a suitable material such as silk, organza or sprigged muslin. The material may be embroidered or pleated depending on whether it is to be used for male or female clothing.

Bath Bags

This last idea was given to me during a trip to Australia where lavender has been grown ever since it was introduced to the country by some of the early settlers. The lavender bath bag has a dual purpose: it can be used instead of soap and is also very good for the skin. The ingredients are three cups of rolled oats which are sprinkled with twenty drops of lavender oil and then sewn into a small gauze sachet. Alternatively, pile the lavender-scented oats into a square of muslin and tie up the corners with string to form a purse.

The bag is, however, only really effective for about a week, after which the contents have to be replenished. The person who gave me the details added that her teenage daughter, who hated using ordinary soap on her skin, claimed that the bath bag kept her completely free of pimples.

Chapter 7
An A–Z of Lavender Cures

Lavender has been used medicinally since the days of Ancient Greece and probably even earlier than that. The first man known to have compiled a list of plants and their medicinal uses was the Greek physician Pedanius Dioscorides, from Anazarb in Cilicia, who lived during the first century AD and wrote a great work on *materia medica*. In this he recorded that the first lavender to be known widely and used in medicine was *Lavandula stoechas*. His book remained the standard work until as late as the sixteenth century, when the herbalist John Gerard (1545–1612) produced his influential *Herball* in 1597. Gerard, who kept Lord Burghley's gardens for over twenty years, where he undoubtedly learned a great deal about the healing properties of plants and herbs, unhesitatingly prescribed lavender for all those with a 'light migrain or swimming of the braine'. His cure? To bathe the temples with lavender water until the pain disappeared.

Just how well established was the use of lavender as a curative can be gauged by the references to it in many other works of medicine and learning. It even found its way into literary fiction – *vide* that famous reference in Jane Austen's classic, *Sense and Sensibility* (1811): 'some lavender drops which she was at length persuaded to take were of use'.

Although it is surprising that so little scientific research has been conducted into the nature of lavender's curative powers, an interesting experiment was carried out in the summer of 1995 at the Hinchingbrooke Hospital at Huntingdon in Cambridgeshire, to test the effectiveness of the essential oil in preventing discomfort in women after childbirth. Inspired by the traditional belief that the antiseptic and healing properties of lavender oil in a bath would help women after giving birth, researchers undertook a blind randomised clinical trial using 635 postnatal women. The patients were divided into three groups: the first were given pure lavender oil, the second a synthetic lavender oil, and the third an inert substance. The 'oils' were then used daily for the ten days immediately after birth to see if they would reduce perineal discomfort.

When the discomfort scores were later collected and analysed, the results revealed that those women using pure lavender oil recorded lower scores on the third and fifth days – the days on which a mother is usually discharged home and her perineal discomfort is high. While the researchers were not prepared to conclude that the lavender oil did significantly reduce postnatal discomfort, 'there is evidence to suggest that lavender oil used in the bath may help alleviate discomfort at certain times.' The study urged more research and added that as no side-effects had been found, 'it seems that lavender oil may be a useful additional remedy to complement other forms of treatment helping postnatal mothers.'

In the following pages I have collected a number of similar treatments utilising lavender which have been in common currency for varying periods of time, some for centuries and others of more recent origin. It is, however, important for the reader to be aware that although lavender is believed by a growing number of people to be as effective as, if not more than, some orthodox forms of medication in dealing with a variety of minor physical and mental ailments, there is NO substitute for immediately consulting a doctor or qualified medical practitioner if the condition seems serious. The cures here are merely suggestions of ways in which minor physical and mental conditions might be prevented or the discomfort made easier to bear with the aid of the medicinal herb.

Acne

This unsightly skin condition, which often afflicts adolescents, is caused by an inflammation of the sebaceous glands. Sebum is a natural oil that lubricates the skin, and if secreted in excess of the skin's need builds up in hair follicles and oily areas around the nose and chin. Spots occur when the sebum becomes trapped under the skin. Lavender is good for regulating the production of sebum, and the essential oil, which acts as an antiseptic and healer, can be applied directly to swollen pustules. Mixed with wheatgerm oil, lavender will soothe and help promote new cell growth, with the wheatgerm minimising any scarring. Use one drop of lavender to one tablespoon of wheatgerm oil, and apply the mixture gently once daily. Do not squeeze the spots, and ensure that the essential oil does not get into the eyes.

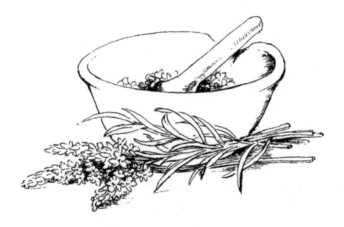

An apothecary's bowl can be very useful in preparing lavender for medicinal use (*Pip Miller*).

Arthritis

Elderly people have for hundreds of years looked to lavender to ease the pain and stiffness caused by osteoarthritis, an inflammation of the joints. Because it is an anti-inflammatory, lavender may be used in baths, compresses and massages. In the bath, up to ten drops of the essential oil may be used on their own; or, alternatively, three drops of lavender and four each of lemon and rosemary. To make a compress, add five drops each of lavender and camomile to two pints of cold water into which a flannel is placed for soaking. A recommended mixture for use in massaging the joints is five drops each of lavender, lemon, coriander and cajuput blended with 50 ml (2 fl oz) of a base oil.

Asthma

This problem, which causes wheezing and difficulty in breathing, can be helped by inhaling a mixture of oils including lavender. As an inhalant, five drops each of lavender, peppermint and eucalyptus are suggested; while if the same three oils are to be used in an essence burner, ten drops of each are recommended. Regular treatment is considered important in both cases.

Athlete's Foot

A fungal growth which is first indicated by thickened, moist skin between the toes. To prevent the skin becoming itchy, dry and eventually peeling off, a footbath or compress of lavender oil, which has anti-fungal powers, is recommended. Place the feet in a bowl of warm water into which two drops each of lavender, tagetes and tea tree have been poured. Soak for ten minutes each evening and dry carefully. Alternatively, last thing at night apply a warm compress containing the same mixture of essential oils to the infected foot, cover with clingfilm, and place in a sock overnight.

Blisters

Lavender is widely held to be a good *preventative* of blisters on the feet rather than a cure. One course of action is to add two drops of the essential oil to stockings or socks which are going to be used in strenuous activity; or a few of the plant's leaves or flowers put in the footwear will have the same effect. Both treatments can also be used in new shoes when they are being worn in, to prevent blisters from developing.

Blood Pressure

Although the best advice is to have your blood pressure checked regularly by a doctor, lavender has long been accepted as a means of encouraging relaxation in order to prevent hypertension. You have the option of using mixtures of the essential oil in either a bath or for massage. In the bath, an ideal mixture is four drops of lavender oil, and three each of ylang ylang and clary sage. For a massage: mix five drops each of lavender, ylang ylang and melissa to 50 ml (2 fl oz) of a base lotion and rub onto the chest, abdomen and soles of the feet before going to bed.

Boils

A hot compress using lavender oil can help in treating these swellings of pus which appear on various parts of the body. To a hot, damp flannel add five drops each of lavender, camomile and tea tree and apply the compress to the inflamed area twice a day, ideally in the morning and evening. The stated quantities should not be exceeded and if the boil gets larger medical advice should be sought.

Bruises

Bruising is caused by the breaking of small blood vessels just beneath the surface of the skin, and those who bruise easily are recommended to add a mixture of five drops each of lavender oil and cypress to their bath-water on a regular basis to help strengthen the blood vessels. To treat a bruise, apply several drops of the essential oil to the damaged part and follow with a cold compress. This will help ease the pain and bring out the injury.

Bunions

People who suffer from these deformities of the big toe joint must, of course, choose their footwear with care, but if a bunion becomes inflamed it can be treated by a massage oil in which lavender plays an important part. To a tablespoonful of a suitable carrier oil add a drop of lavender oil and then gently rub the bunion with this for at least five minutes. A daily massage with this mixture is recommended for lasting relief.

Burns

Serious burns require immediate medical attention, but for smaller lesions lavender oil can be a great comfort. Plunging the injured part under cold water is one immediate course of action, but if neat lavender oil is to hand, apply two to three drops which will help ease the pain as well as preventing blistering. This application should be repeated hourly until the discomfort has ceased.

Cold Sores

For generations these unsightly little blemishes which form around the mouth have been cured by country folk with an application of lavender oil. Using a small ball of cotton wool, dab the cold sore with two to three drops of the essential oil first thing in the morning and last thing at night. Repeat until the spot has disappeared.

Colds and Flu

One of the commonest of all ailments, the cold is caused by a virus infection of the upper respiratory tract, producing coughs, sneezes and congestion of the nose and throat. Lavender oil is a prophylactic – that is it can help prevent colds and flu – as well as being able to give a boost to the immune system. It is, however, important to take action as soon as the first signs of a developing cold become evident, by using steam inhalation or an essence burner. Up to ten drops of lavender may be used in the burner, or half that in an inhalation with a hot water base. Some people prefer a blending of lavender, lemon and tea tree; while others swear that the best recipe is a hot bath to which five drops each of lavender and tea tree have been added. In the case of a viral infection that leads to influenza, the doctor should be called.

Constipation

An uncomfortable and unpleasant condition affecting the bowels, for which a lavender massage may provide the answer. Prepare a mixture of five drops each of lavender, rosemary, fennel and black pepper in 50 ml (2 fl oz) of a base oil. Massage this onto the abdomen in a clockwise direction to stimulate the internal muscles into contracting and relaxing. Repeat morning and evening for a week. If there is no improvement after this time, a doctor should be consulted.

Cuts and Grazes

Minor injuries such as cuts and grazes can be soothed and helped to mend by the application of drops of lavender oil applied with a swab of cotton wool. It may be advisable to cover the wound with a plaster afterwards, but in any event the use of lavender will heal the injury with notable speed.

Dandruff

The fine, dry, powdery flakes that indicate dandruff in the hair and which are often brought about by stress, are best combatted by the soothing power of oil of lavender. Prepare a mixture of five drops each of lavender and geranium, two drops of sandalwood and 30 ml (1½ fl oz) of base oil. Apply this all over the scalp to wet hair and leave for a minimum of two hours. Then use a mild, unperfumed shampoo and rinse thoroughly. Give the hair a final rinse by adding the same blend of essential oils to a jug of warm water – mix well before applying. Repeat the treatment every day, decreasing to twice a week as the symptoms improve. To make another preparation which will provide a complete course of treatment, take six drops each of lavender and cedarwood, three drops of camomile, three teaspoonsful of cider vinegar and 300 ml ($^1/_2$ pt) of distilled water. Pour the distilled water into a bottle (preferably one made of dark glass), then add the cider vinegar and essential oils. Always shake the bottle well and use as for the previous treatment, applying sufficient to wet the hair thoroughly.

Depression

Depression – that feeling of apathy, loss of appetite, irregular sleep and generally low spirits – calls for an oil that is both normalising and uplifting, and lavender comes highly recommended. The best treatment is a back massage which will obviously have to involve a partner who can also talk you through your troubles at the same time. The massage oil should be made of two drops each of lavender and geranium and one of camomile, mixed with 15 ml (3 teaspoons) of base oil. This should be gently worked into the whole of the back from the shoulders to the base of the spine, and repeated twice daily until the gloom lifts. In the case of depressive illness seek medical advice.

Diarrhoea

There is a variety of proprietary medicines on sale for loose bowels – but if the condition has been brought about by anxiety of any sort, then a lavender mixture will help ease the symptoms. To five drops of lavender add the same amounts of peppermint, camomile and sandalwood in a 25 ml (1 fl oz) base and apply this in a warm compress to the abdominal area. Some experts suggest that a compress consisting solely of lavender oil can be even more effective.

Eczema

This skin disorder with symptoms of dry, itchy or weeping skin may be hereditary or else brought about by stress. In serious cases medical help is essential, but where the inflammation is annoying rather than painful, a lavender compress or massage will help heal the eczema. The compress should be cold and should contain a mixture of two drops each of lavender and camomile plus one of geranium. Dab this gently onto the affected parts. Where the skin is actually weeping, a mixture of four drops each of lavender and evening primrose plus two of camomile in a 30 ml (1¹/₂ fl oz) base should be applied each morning and night. Extra virgin olive oil is highly recommended as the base.

Fibrositis

The shoulders are the area of the body most likely to be affected by fibrositis and best treated in a lavender bath. To warm rather than hot water add four drops of lavender and three each of camomile and cajuput. Then lie back with the shoulders beneath the surface and soak for half an hour.

Flatulence

Indigestion is generally caused by eating too much and/or too quickly, or by subsisting on a poor diet. However, the discomfort flatulence causes can be eased by lavender which is an acknowledged aid to digestion. To two drops each of lavender and caraway, add four of peppermint in 15 ml (3 teaspoons) of a base oil. This should be gently applied to either the upper or lower abdomen depending on where the discomfort is felt to originate. If the flatulence gets progressively worse, medical advice should be sought in case there is a more serious problem, like gallstones or a peptic ulcer.

Foot Cream

For those who suffer from rough, dry skin on the feet, there is a lavender and beeswax mix which will not only provide relief, but used regularly will help to improve the condition. The ingredients are two tablespoons of white beeswax granules (these are preferable to the solid blocks of beeswax which have to be grated to melt quickly), two tablespoons of cocoa butter and six tablespoons of apricot kernel oil. You will also need ten drops each of lavender, rosemary and sage oil, plus 15 drops of evening primrose. Melt the beeswax and cocoa butter in a small bowl or container over a pan of boiling water, stirring gently until the wax is completely dissolved. Warm the apricot oil in another utensil, and then pour into the mixture, stirring all the while. Once this mixture is consistent, remove it from any source of heat and add the essential oils. Finally, the foot cream should be poured into small jars and stored in a cool, dark place to keep fresh and ready for use. This cream is said to be most effective if rubbed into the feet immediately after they have been bathed.

Gout

This complaint, which causes the feet to swell, has for years been associated in popular belief with drinking too much port! In fact the inflammation, caused by an excess of uric acid in the blood, is just as likely to affect the hands as the feet, and can strike the young as well as the old. A massage oil is recommended, consisting of five drops each of lavender and juniper berry added to ten drops of camomile. Ideally the mixture should be applied to the affected part of the body twice a day. Where it is the feet only that are affected by the gout, some experts recommend a warm foot bath into which three drops each of lavender and juniper berry and four of camomile are stirred.

Hair Loss

Alopecia – either temporary baldness or sudden hair loss – can be caused by physical or emotional stress. A consultation with a doctor when it occurs is certainly very important, but lavender oil, which is said to stimulate hair growth, can help the recovery process. Prepare a mixture of two drops each of lavender and thyme oil with equal quantities of jojoba and almond oils. Massage this into the scalp and then cover the head with a warm towel for at least an hour. Repeat this process three times a week until an improvement is noticed.

Hay Fever

This allergy affects a great many people and can become a problem from the moment the first tree pollens appear, right through the summer months. In country districts men and women have for generations carried handkerchiefs spotted with two drops of lavender oil, or alternatively with a sprig of lavender contained in the folds, to sniff whenever the need arises to clear the nasal passages.

Headaches

Headaches, of course, come in many different forms and may affect different areas of the head, but lavender can play a part in relieving the pain in various ways. The simplest method of easing a general headache is to put two drops of lavender oil on your forefinger and rub it across your temples, around the outer corners of the eye bone, behind the ears and then across the back of the neck. Repeat this process twice. A massage of three drops each of lavender and eucalyptus in 15 ml (3 teaspoons) of base oil can be used for the same process, but if it is applied by another person it can also include the shoulders and lower neck and will have an even more beneficial effect. Two drops of lavender oil on a tissue, mixed with the same amounts of sweet marjoram and peppermint, make a good inhaler for tackling migraines. Soaking in a hot bath into which three drops each of lavender, camomile and sweet marjoram have been added will help to lift a tension headache. Two or three drops of lavender oil on the edges of a pillow can help if you go to bed with a headache – although if the symptoms persist or grow more severe, do seek medical advice.

Head Lice

These small insects which infest the scalp and feed by sucking blood from the skin are most common in children, and lavender oil is one of the herb insecticides that can be used to help relieve the condition. A recommended rinse for use on youngsters can be made by putting 74 ml (3 fl oz) of vegetable oil into a bottle and adding 15 drops of lavender and five drops each of geranium and eucalyptus. Shake the mixture well before use, applying it to wet hair and massaging it thoroughly into the scalp. Do pay particular attention to the areas around the ears and the nape of the neck where the lice breed. (Also take care that the oil mix does not get into the child's eyes.) Leave the mixture on for at least an hour before shampooing thoroughly. The process should be repeated daily until the lice and eggs have disappeared.

Insomnia

Anxiety and tension are among the primary causes of sleepless nights – not to mention over-excitement or eating the wrong foods. Lavender has long been credited with sedative and calming properties. A highly recommended sleeping blend consists of three drops each of lavender and ylang ylang and two of camomile mixed in 15 ml (3 teaspoons) of base lotion. This can either be added to a warm bath about an hour before going to bed or can be massaged into the face and shoulders. Three drops of lavender and two of camomile on a tissue make an excellent inhalant – breathe deeply three times – or instead put two or three drops of lavender oil on either side of the pillow or the sheets and inhale deeply several times before settling down. Result . . . Zzzz.

Lumbago

Massages or baths containing lavender oil are popular remedies for this painful condition which affects the muscles and ligaments of the lower back. A suitable oil which can be worked in gently by a partner consists of eight drops each of lavender, black pepper and cajuput in a 50 ml (2 fl oz) base. This should be applied twice daily and always in a warm room, as heat helps to ease lumbago. For a soothing bath, add five drops each of lavender and camomile to the water which should be as hot as you can comfortably bear.

Menstrual Problems

Women discovered centuries ago that certain herbs could help them through their monthly cycles if used between two and ten days before the onset of a period. The application of a lavender-based oil massage around the navel is very soothing and balancing emotion-ally and will help encourage the flow. The mix should consist of four drops each of lavender and clary sage with two drops of melissa added to 30 ml (1½ fl oz) of base oil. Ideally, this blend should be applied twice daily for up to ten days before the period is due. Women who suffer from irregular periods should daily rub onto the abdomen and small of the back a mixture of two drops each of lavender, rose and clary sage with three drops of camomile in a 30 ml (1½ fl oz) base. This will help re-establish the hormonal balance.

Migraine

The unexpected migraine is a very unpleasant experience which can affect the vision and even bring on nausea. Lavender is one of the essential oils recommended in the treatment, although it is only fair to point out that the sense of smell can sometimes be so heightened in certain people that even the smell of lavender may be upsetting. If this is not the case, then a mixture of three drops each of lavender and cajuput and four of lemon in an essence burner and gently inhaled will bring gradual relief.

Mouth Ulcers

Mouth ulcers usually appear on the gums, inside the cheeks or along the edge of the tongue and are caused by stress or stomach upsets. Lavender is one of the essential oils that has anti-fungal properties and is best taken in a mouthwash to cure the complaint. Add one drop each of lavender, geranium and tea tree to half a glass of water and gargle with this three times a day. **Do not swallow the solution.**

Muscle Cramp

Usually caused by over-exercise when the muscles have been deprived of oxygenated blood. Massage is obviously good for muscles to keep the blood flowing, but a sudden muscle cramp or spasm can be eased by rubbing on a mixture of five drops each of lavender, cajuput, marjoram and camomile added to a 50 ml (2 fl oz) base. Sportsmen and women are well advised to keep a supply of this mixture to hand for use after any particularly strenuous competition.

Nappy Rash

Aromatherapists have discovered what country mums knew for generations: that this painful red rash can be cured by lavender, which has the ability to heal broken skin through stimulating cell renewal. The following mix is widely recommended for babies and can be applied when the nappy is being changed: four drops of lavender, two drops of camomile, one drop of sandalwood in a 60 ml (2½ fl oz) base of oil or lotion. When washing nappies in a washing machine, add six drops of lavender oil to the softening agent in the rinse programme as this will also lessen the chance of nappy rash.

Nausea

The feeling of wanting to be sick can be caused by any number of reasons, but essential oils like lavender, camomile, basil and peppermint have a sedative quality which can help overcome this sensation. One widely used method of treating nausea is to sprinkle three drops each of lavender and peppermint onto a tissue or handkerchief and, sitting quietly and still, inhale deeply three times.

Palpitations

A variety of emotions can cause the heart to flutter or beat more forcefully, and a soothing essential oil will help to calm the person down. Lavender is ideal and can be used as an inhalant, a massage or in a relaxing bath. To inhale, put three drops of lavender, ylang ylang and neroli on a tissue and breathe deeply. For a massage, get your partner to rub into the areas around your heart and solar plexus a mix of eight drops of lavender and ylang ylang and four of melissa in 50 ml (2 fl oz) of base oil. If a bath seems more suitable, then add to the water five drops each of lavender, ylang ylang and melissa. However, if the palpitations persist it may be a sign of high blood pressure or a heart problem and medical advice should be sought.

Phlebitis

Lavender oil in a compress is suggested for this leg inflammation. To a flannel dampened with cold water add five drops each of lavender, lemon and camomile which should then be placed on the afflicted part of the leg and left for as long as possible. Under no circumstances should the leg be massaged.

Piles

Referred to in medical terms as haemorrhoids, these often painful, bleeding veins in the lower rectum require professional advice, but the condition can be made more comfortable with lavender oil. Make up a mixture consisting of five drops each of lavender and lemon and ten of cypress in 15 ml (3 teaspoons) of a bland oil base. Apply with cotton wool first thing in the morning and last thing at night for a soothing effect.

Rheumatism

Rheumatism affects the muscles rather than the joints and is generally brought on after getting cold and wet or sitting in a draught. Lavender is good at relaxing muscles and relieving pain and can be used in either a massage or a bath mixture. One particular massage oil, which combines calming and anti-inflammatory elements, consists of five drops each of lavender, eucalyptus, camomile and juniper berry mixed with 60 ml (2 fl oz) of base oil. This should be rubbed *gently* onto the inflamed area. The bath formula consists of two drops each of lavender and rosemary and three of eucalyptus sprinkled into the warm water.

Sinusitis

An inflammation of the nasal passage which can be brought about by tobacco smoke, foggy weather, stress or as a direct result of a heavy cold. Lavender is at the core of a decongestant lotion made from three drops of lavender, two of peppermint and four of eucalyptus diluted in 15 ml (3 teaspoons) of base lotion. This should be rubbed gently into the face around the area of the nose each night. An inhalation of lavender (one drop), peppermint (one drop) and eucalyptus (two drops), sprinkled onto a tissue and breathed in deeply three times each morning and night, has also been found to be very beneficial.

Sore Feet

This is an old country tip originally said to have been devised by women who had spent long hours in the fields at harvest time. When they arrived home they had terribly sore feet and at once plunged them into a bowl of warm water to which had been added some lavender flowers, a little sage and thyme, and a teaspoon of salt. Half an hour in this mixture and your feet – like those of the good ladies of old – should be completely rejuvenated.

Sore Throat

Whether caused by an infection or by inhaling smoke or dust, a gargle mix containing lavender oil is recommended for curing a sore throat. First fill a cup with warm water and stir in a teaspoon of honey. Then add two drops each of lavender, tea tree and lemon oils, stirring well. Gargle thoroughly **without swallowing** until all the mixture is finished. Some aromatherapists also recommend massaging the throat area with a mixture of eight drops each of lavender, bergamot and tea tree mixed in a 50 ml (2 fl oz) base.

Sprains

These usually occur from over-exertion, when ligaments are torn or stretched. Unless there is a chance that a bone may have been broken – in which case seek medical advice at once – a lavender compress and lots of rest are the best cure. To a cold compress add three drops of lavender which is calming, and four each of sweet marjoram and rosemary which are analgesics, mixed together in 15 ml (3 teaspoons) of base oil. Never massage a sprain, but do repeat the compress treatment until the pain and swelling have gone.

Stress

Lavender features in many cures when stress is a contributory factor, but the most important thing of all is to try to relax, take plenty of exercise and maybe even seek professional advice. A quick relief for sudden stress is to stop whatever you are doing, sprinkle four drops of lavender on a tissue and inhale deeply. There is another formula of relaxing blends which can be added to a warm bath or else used in a full-body massage given by a friend or partner. It consists of two drops each of lavender, sandalwood, geranium and one of ylang ylang. For the massage, the oils must be blended with 15 ml (3 teaspoons) of base oil.

Sunburn

There are many brands of suntan lotion on the market and a wealth of warnings and advice, but still people persist in spending too long sunbathing, with the inevitable consequence of sore red patches all over their bodies. One of the simplest and quickest antidotes is neat lavender oil which should be dabbed onto the reddened skin with cotton wool to ease the pain and prevent blisters. Aromatherapists recommend careful exposure to the sun and the use of a sun-screen oil blended from two drops each of lavender and camomile with 20 ml (4 teaspoons) of sesame oil and 30 ml (6 teaspoons) of coconut oil. An after-sun lotion which can be beneficial, whether skin has been burnt or not, is a mixture of six drops each of lavender and bergamot with five drops each of sandalwood and camomile in 50 ml (2 fl oz) of base oil. If sunstroke is suspected, get immediate medical help for the victim; meanwhile apply a cold, wet compress dabbed with two drops of lavender oil to the back of the neck and forehead.

Toothache

The pain from a decayed tooth cries out for only one solution: a visit to the dentist as quickly as possible. In the interim, two to three drops of neat lavender oil applied to the aching tooth will help ease the pain. **Be careful not to swallow the oil.**

Warts

Ignoring the old folk custom of attempting to remove warts by 'charming', many country people believe that lavender provides a more practical solution to these unsightly skin blemishes. Using neat lavender oil, put two drops on the wart three times a day and continue until the condition improves.

Chapter 8
Useful Tips with Lavender

The versatility of lavender extends into many different areas of daily life and in this chapter I have brought together some of the most useful hints and tips that have been passed on to me by friends and acquaintances over the years. Some of these ideas bear all the hallmarks of centuries-old use, while others are clearly much more recent. Not a few, I suspect, will still have much to offer for centuries to come.

Air Freshener

Lavender has been described as one of the best air fresheners, and in its basic form is one of most inexpensive. A bunch of lavender hung in the kitchen, bathroom or lavatory, for example, has long been said to be good at removing odours and imparting a gentle, pleasant fragrance. During the Middle Ages lavender and other herbs were strewn throughout buildings to mask unsavoury smells, but although this is hardly practicable today, there is no reason why a generous layer of dried lavender flowers should not be placed under doormats or between the underlay and a carpet. Alternatively, pop a few drops of lavender oil into a bowl of very hot water and this will evaporate and fill any room with fragrant perfume. The same effect can be achieved by two drops of oil dropped onto a purpose-made ceramic 'aromatherapy ring', which sits on the light bulb of a table lamp. Stalks of lavender in a flower arrangement will also keep a room smelling fresh – 'Hidcote' is said to be the most suitable variety – and a few sprigs of the plant thrown onto the ashes of a fire last thing at night will clear away the smell of soot by the following morning.

Ant Guard

Although ants are known to like sweet things, they have a strong dislike of lavender, which can be used to your advantage. The herb has its own built-in safetyguard to keep ants away from the nectar that attracts bees and enables them to pollinate the plant. With this in mind, use the cheaper form of lavender oil as a spray for getting rid of ants inside the house or even in the garden where they have a habit of making their presence felt on patios and paved areas.

Clothes Wash

Lavender is thought to have got its name from the Latin lavare, 'to wash', and has been used for centuries in laundries for washing and rinsing linen. Indeed, it may well have been a component in the wood-ash mixtures which preceded soaps and detergents. Although most of us now use washing machines for getting our clothes clean, lavender can still be of use. To ensure that your wash is thoroughly clean add three drops each of lavender and geranium to the final rinsing water, or else mix the blend with your softening agent in the rinse compartment of your machine. Finally, you might like to know that for generations the traditional place to spread out clean washing to dry has been on lavender bushes where they can be further impregnated by the scent of the plant.

First Aid Kit

Lavender oil, as a natural antiseptic and healer, should be an essential item in any household first aid kit. Obviously people have different opinions as to what should form a basic kit, but I would recommend including the following: several large and small bandages, plasters, adhesive tape, cotton wool, gauze, a piece of cotton cloth to be used in compresses, and pairs of scissors and tweezers. The essential oils you should not be without are lavender, geranium, tea tree, camomile and sweet marjoram. It is important to keep this kit out of the reach of children, and where an injury is at all serious use the oils only as a stand-by while medical help is sought.

Flies

The common housefly is one of the curses of everyday living, whether your home is in town or country, but a combination of lavender and mint was claimed by the writers of the old herbals to be good at deterring these insects. The lavender flowers and mint sprigs should be used in arrangements such as posies or bouquets, and put in the areas where flies are most prevalent, like kitchens and lavatories. Country folk still refer quaintly to these creations as 'fly-away posies'.

Disinfectant

An effective disinfectant which is ideal for sinks and baths can be made from lavender as a natural alternative to chemical disinfectants. Place as many leaves and flowering stems as you can get into your largest pan and boil for thirty minutes. Use as little water as possible because this will make the resulting disinfectant more concentrated. Strain and then apply the liquid on a cloth to the appropriate surfaces. Friends who have used this mixture say that the addition of a little washing-up liquid helps to get rid of any grease from surfaces. The lavender disinfectant should be stored in a very cool place – ideally a fridge – and used within seven days of being made because after this time it begins to lose its strength. A few drops of lavender oil added to hot water will provide a general disinfectant when you are cleaning down walls or washing floors. A sprinkling of oil in the sink, drainage pipe and lavatory bowl will also help as part of household hygiene.

Handbags

Fashionable ladies in Victorian England used to keep blocks of compressed lavender in their handbags and purses so that a sweet smell greeted them whenever they were opened. Some even had the linings of their muffs stuffed with dried lavender – which perhaps explains what were assumed to be coy glances from behind their mittens. They were more likely surreptitious sniffs of the invigo-rating lavender! Today the same idea can still be utilised in handbags and purses – or even the inside of ladies' gloves – with equal effect.

Hangover

If you have dined or celebrated a little too well and woken up with a throbbing head, then a lavender massage may help you to overcome the pain. Mix five drops of lavender oil with three of peppermint and geranium in a base of sweet almond. Then ask your partner to massage the mixture *slowly* and *gently* into the base of your neck. After half an hour you should feel a lot better, and the fragrance still floating around the room should certainly be beneficial, too. Gardening expert Adrienne Wild says that the best drink she knows to beat a hangover is an infusion of lavender. Her recipe requires you to put three sprigs of lavender into a pot of tea, strain, and then drink without the addition of milk or sugar.

Insect Bites and Stings

Because lavender repels many insects, the oil extracted from it can help to soothe and heal any of their unwelcome attacks. It is important first to remove the sting of a bee, if it still in the flesh, before beginning treatment. The most widely recommended curative is a mixture of a drop each of lavender and tea tree applied to the inflamed area. This should be repeated at hourly intervals until the irritation stops.

Jet Lag

After a long flight, the sensation of jet lag can be overcome by using lavender oil. To a moist flannel or pad add five drops of the essential oil and massage this into the feet and ankles in an upward direction. This cure came to me highly recommended by an air hostess who regularly had to make trips to the Far East and Australia.

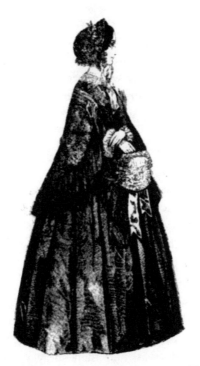

A Victorian gentlewoman with lavender-scented hand muff
(*The Lady's Newspaper*, 1853).

Mosquito Deterrent

Mosquitoes and a number of other flying insects appear to be repelled by lavender. A mixture of lavender oil with a carrier oil of your choice will produce an aromatic liquid which can be applied to any exposed parts of the body to keep off these marauding creatures. When abroad in hot climates, use this at night in conjunction with a few drops of lavender oil in an oil burner and you should be guaranteed a restful and insect-free slumber. Country people say that a bowl of lavender-scented pot-pourri put near a window or door will also stop mosquitoes from entering the house.

Needlework

For at least two hundred years needlewomen have known the value of putting dried lavender in their pincushions or needlecases to release a delicious fragrance whenever they are being used. The oil still remaining in the flowers has the added advantage of preventing the pins and needles from going rusty.

Pets

Lavender oil can be used quite safely on household pets such as cats and dogs. In the case of a wound or abscess, add three drops of lavender to 300 ml ($^{1}/_{2}$ pint) water which has been boiled and then allowed to cool. Bathe the afflicted part of the animal with a cloth. Fleas can also be a problem to domestic animals, and the following cure was given to me by an aromatherapist who specialises in dealing with pets. Pour 30 ml ($1^{1}/_{2}$ fl oz) of water into a spray container and add two drops each of lavender and tea tree and six drops of geranium. Shake the mixture well, ruffle up the animal's fur around the infested areas, and then spray gently. My informant suggested that it is a good idea to let the cat or dog sniff the mixture first to allay its fears – it smells very pleasant; and it is also advisable to have someone else present to hold the pet and shield its eyes before beginning to spray. A little dried lavender put in a pet's basket will help to keep fleas away.

Scented Notepaper

Although scented notepaper can be purchased at many stationers, it is not difficult to give ordinary paper that unmistakable fragrance of lavender. Just sprinkle the paper with lavender oil (it will not leave a mark) and store the sheets in a box into which you have popped some dried lavender flowers. The combination of the aroma and your loving words can make this a most effective kind of correspondence!

Tea Cosy

My grandmother, who always had a garden full of lavender, used to put a fresh sprig into the padding of her tea cosy every year so that whenever she made a pot the heat from the brew would release the most delightful scent to accompany the pleasure of her cuppa. I have been told that some cooks do exactly the same thing with their oven gloves.

Washing-up

Although this may not be one of the favourite chores, if you still do the dishes and cutlery by hand, then adding a little lavender oil will ensure that they are clean and free from germs. Sprinkle two drops each of lavender and geranium oils into the water and the herbs will exercise their antiseptic properties although, sadly, such a small amount will not be enough to create an aroma while you work.

Window-cleaning

Grimy windows which do not come really clean with soapy water may well respond better if lavender vinegar is used. Dampen a cloth with the vinegar and rub vigorously. Remember to leave a trace of the lavender vinegar in the corners of the frames as this will create a pleasant smell after you have finished. A method of making lavender vinegar which is especially good at this task is to fill a jar with lavender, some lemon verbena and mint leaves and pour on hot vinegar. This mixture must be left for three days before it is ready for use, and although the colour will initially be purple, this will gradually fade and certainly leave no traces on any surface.

Wood Polish

For several hundred years lavender has been an ingredient in a furniture polish which can be used on either light or dark wood. The ingredients required are 450 ml (16 fl oz) of beeswax and the same volumes of turpentine and of olive oil or linseed oil (olive oil is ideal for light woods and linseed for darker ones). Put the mixture into a pan and heat, adding four sprigs of lavender flowers. **Caution: These are highly flammable ingredients, and should not be heated over an open flame. Use a double-boiler and heat only enough to melt the beeswax.** When it becomes liquid, take out the lavender because it has done its job. Finally, pour into several jars and allow to set. The polish should be ready for use the next day. This makes over 1 litre (2 pints) of polish, so you might consider giving some away as gifts.

Lavender oil is a traditional ingredient in some of the better quality polishes sold commercially for fine wooden furniture and parquet floors. Even everyday tins of polish can, however, be improved by adding a few drops of the essential oil to the cream or wax, though it will probably be necessary to warm the container to allow the lavender to mix with the rest of the contents.

Chapter 9
Cooking with Lavender

Surprising though it may seem, lavender has been used in cooking for centuries, with medieval monks being among the earliest to apply it to the culinary arts. Since then housewives and chefs all over the world have discovered that there is more to the herb than just its beauty and perfume. With careful use it can add a unique flavour and aroma to a whole variety of dishes, ranging from those served at breakfast right through to the evening meal.

The passing years have demonstrated that lavender actually deserves the same kind of recognition in the culinary world as that already enjoyed by a number of other herbs more usually associated with cooking – rosemary, sage, thyme and dill – and its presence as an ingredient in even just one course can add considerably to the enjoyment of the meal as a whole.

As a general rule, the flowers of the lavender have a stronger flavour than the leaves. And when it comes to using the herb in any dish it is important – as any good cook will tell you when trying something new – to be flexible and ready to experiment while searching for the most suitable blend of ingredients. I can promise you that lavender will repay its diligent use in cooking with some great taste sensations!

Breakfast

Lavender can be used in each of the three items which for me make up the traditional breakfast – a cup of tea, a slice of bread (toasted if you prefer) and marmalade. Here are my favourite recipes for each.

Lavender Tea

A tasty brew of lavender will put you in an upbeat frame of mind for the day. It is a good idea to experiment with the amount of dried lavender flowers you use, but I would suggest 5 ml (1 teaspoon) of the flowers per cup (227 ml or 8 oz) of boiling water as a trial cuppa. If the flavour appeals to you, then make your lavender tea in a teapot just as you would a normal brew, allowing it to stand for a few minutes before pouring. Some people even sweeten the tea with a little clear honey.

A brew which mixes lavender and lime flowers is said to be very good at calming people and relieving tension. The yellow, scented flowers of the lime (linden) tree – not the citrus fruit tree – bloom in July and can be dried and stored in the same way as lavender. Like dried lavender, they can also be bought from a herbalist. To brew this tea in a pot, allow 5 ml (1 teaspoon) each of the lavender and lime for 2 cups (450 ml or 16 fl oz). The lavender and lime tea should be allowed to stand for 6–8 minutes before being poured through a strainer. Again, sweeten with clear honey if desired.

Although both the above can be served at tea-time – or any other hour of the day for that matter – the ideal brew at the end of a tiring and difficult day is a mixture of three herbal flowers and China green tea. In a teapot mix one part each of dried lavender and dried camomile flowers with a half part of dried yarrow flowers and one part China green tea. Add boiling water and allow to stand for about three minutes. A friend who is especially fond of this brew says that it is very good for easing tension headaches and migraines, and she always refers to it as my 'headache tea'. (You might also like to try adding two or three heads of dried lavender to your tea caddy in order to give the tea a gently scented aroma.)

Barley and Lavender Loaf

This is a traditional English bread, originally created by monks who used honey collected from the bees that clustered on their lavender bushes. The bread is said to be particularly nourishing for those who spend long, busy days at work, like the original monks. The ingredients required are:

510 g (1 lb 2 oz) strong wholemeal flour
225 g (8 oz) barley flour
25 g (1 oz) rice flour
$^1/_2$ tablespoon salt
15 g ($^1/_2$ oz) fresh yeast
60 ml (2$^1/_2$ fl oz) brown ale
water (as specified)
2 teaspoons clear lavender honey

To prepare: Mix the dry ingredients in a warmed bowl. Blend the yeast to a cream with the ale, mix 1$^1/_2$ cups/350 ml/12 fl oz of warm water with the lavender honey. Stir the mixture into the dry ingredients and work into a firm dough, adding extra warm water as required. When the dough feels elastic, shape it into a ball and remove from the bowl. Next, oil the inside of the bowl lightly. Replace the dough, cover it loosely with oiled polythene, and leave in a warm place until the dough has doubled in bulk. Knock it down with your hands and then shape into two round loaves. Place these in two deep bread tins, mark with a cross-cut, and cover with a cloth until well risen. Pre-heat your oven to Gas 8/230°C/450°F and bake the loaves for about 25 minutes. When cooked, the Barley and Lavender Bread should sound hollow when tapped and it must be allowed to stand until quite cold before cutting.

For those who prefer white bread, I have been told that a delicious lavender-flavoured loaf can be made by using an ordinary bread mix and just topping the dough with a few crumbled dried lavender flowers before putting it in the oven to bake.

Lavender Marmalade

The addition of lavender to marmalade does not, as might be expected, overpower its natural taste and aroma. This recipe was provided for me by the cooks at Norfolk Lavender who also suggested that the Seville oranges may, if necessary, be replaced by ready-prepared canned citrus fruit, but it is important to ensure that there are *no* added preservatives.

1 kg (2 lb 3 oz) Seville oranges
1 lemon
2 litres (3 pts) water
2 kg (4¹/₂ lb) preserving sugar
25 g (1 oz) dried lavender flowers in a muslin bag

To prepare: Cut the oranges and lemon in half, extract the juice and pips, and shred the peel. If the pith is thick remove some. Put the peel, juice and water into a pan, add the pips in a muslin bag and bring to the boil. Simmer gently for approximately 90 minutes (or until you are sure the peel is tender). Squeeze the bag of pips to release any liquid before removing. Stir in the sugar over a gentle heat until it is dissolved. Add the lavender bag and bring to a fast boil for about 10 minutes. Press the juice from the lavender bag. Continue at a fast boil until the setting point is reached (test by putting a teaspoon of the mixture in a saucer and allowing to cool). Leave the marmalade to stand for half an hour, turn into warm, dry jars, and cover with airtight seals.

If you like fresh fruit with your morning meal, then remember that lavender will blend especially well with citrus fruits. Half a grapefruit sprinkled with a few dried lavender flowers is said to change it from being just a breakfast dish to a gastronomic experience!

Lunch and Dinner

There is a whole variety of ways in which lavender can be used in recipes for lunch or dinner meals. The dried flowers, for example, can be used like herbs for seasoning casseroles and stews instead of rosemary or bay leaves; and herring and trout benefit from the addition of little sprigs of the plant before they are grilled. It can be used just as effectively to flavour turkey, chicken and duck in a stuffing made from dried lavender, breadcrumbs and sausagemeat; while joints of meats such as lamb and pork take on a light, spicy aroma with a helping of lavender and redcurrant jelly. Indeed, I suspect that with the growing popularity of lavender it will not be long before one of our more enterprising chefs produces a whole book of recipes! Meanwhile, here are just a few ideas that have been given to me by relatives and friends. By the way, if you are one of those people who enjoy a glass of wine with your meal, try putting a spike of lavender, a slice of cucumber and several pieces of ice into a glass and filling it up with Chablis. Cheers!

Starters

Lavender and Orange Salad

The choice of ingredients for a salad is obviously very much a matter of individual taste. The use of edible flowers in salads is now becoming fashionable again after years of neglect – and those who are startled by the idea should remember that the Romans and the Ancient Chinese ate roses, violets and mallow, among others, and that two of our best-loved vegetables, broccoli and artichokes, are actually the buds of flowers. This said, the flowers of lavender used either fresh or dried can make a pleasing as well as tasty addition to the more traditional salad ingredients. This is a favourite recipe of mine when lavender is in season.

3 ripe oranges
1 teaspoon fresh lavender flowers
1 small Spanish onion
red wine vinegar

To prepare: First slice the oranges, removing the membrane and pith. Chop up the lavender flowers and Spanish onion and place all three ingredients in a bowl. Add three teaspoons of the red wine vinegar, mix gently, and serve.

Dried lavender can also be used on green and mixed salads. When assembling these dishes it is important to handle everything as gently as possible, washing the ingredients carefully and ensuring that they are dry before sprinkling on the lavender to taste. Remember that lavender is very strongly flavoured and should be used sparingly, rather as you would use pepper. Lavender vinegar can add a subtle fragrance to any sort of salad, and I recommend making your own with 600 ml (1 pint) of white wine vinegar and a whole sprig or just some leaves of lavender, about 25 g (1 oz). Put the lavender into a bottle and pour in the vinegar, which has been brought to the boil. Seal the bottle and leave in a cool, dark place for at least two weeks to mature. Before it is ready for the table you will need to remove the wilted lavender, which has now discoloured, and strain into a fresh bottle. Just try a few drops of this on your salads and give your taste-buds a whole new sensation!

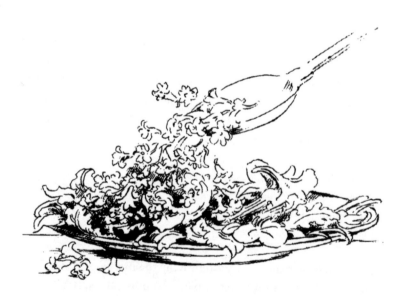

Salad can be made especially delicious with the addition of a little lavender (*Pip Miller*).

Main Courses

Leg of Lamb with Lavender

A popular dish at summer festas and sagras in Europe, especially in Provence and parts of Italy like Nemi in Lazio and Diamante in Calabria, where lavender has been grown for centuries and is held in high regard. In some parts of Europe the leg of a kid is substituted for that of a lamb, but otherwise the recipe is exactly the same. Serves 4.

> 2 large onions
> 2 medium aubergines
> 4 red peppers
> 1 bulb of large-clove garlic
> 1 leg of lamb (approx. 2 kg/ 4^1/$_2$ lb)
> 4 tablespoons extra virgin olive oil
> sprigs of lavender, rosemary, thyme, mint and fennel
> 1 glass *fino* sherry
> salt and pepper

To prepare: First peel and thinly slice the onions, slice the aubergines, and seed and thinly slice the peppers. Leave the garlic cloves whole, but separate and peel them. Next brown the joint all over in two tablespoons of the olive oil. Place the vegetables and garlic in the bottom of a large casserole and lay the meat on top. To this add the herbs, the remainder of the olive oil and the fino sherry and season the whole dish lightly. Place the lid on the casserole, put into an oven preheated to Gas 4/180°C/350°F and cook for 2–2^1/$_2$ hours. Remove the lid for the last 30 minutes. Garnish the joint with fresh herbs before serving. Leg of Lamb with Lavender can also be prepared by putting the joint in a roasting pan and covering it with kitchen foil for part of the cooking time.

Lavender Kebabs

My husband and I first came across Lavender Kebabs some years ago, during a holiday in Morocco (where they are said to have originated). The simple recipe makes them ideal for a barbecue.

chunks of lamb (as appropriate) cut from a leg
lemon juice
25 g (1 oz) dried lavender
vegetables of your choice (suitable for grilling)

To prepare: Use a mortar and pestle to grind up the dried lavender very finely, adding the lemon juice and a little salt as you do so. Then marinate the chunks of lamb in the paste for not less than two hours. Thread the meat on to skewers, alternating with peppers, onions or whatever you choose cut into pieces, and grill to taste on the barbecue. While watching the Lavender Kebabs being prepared in an open-air restaurant in Tangier, we noticed that the cook regularly threw little branches of lavender onto his open fire, which no doubt contributed to the scent and taste of the finished dish which he set before his customers.

Steamed Fish with Lavender Butter

In a number of the fishing communities around the British Isles, housewives still follow a traditional method of preparing steamed fish by cooking it on a rack over boiling water to which a teaspoonful of dried lavender has been added. It gives the most delightful tang to the flavour of the fish. It was in the port of King's Lynn that I collected the following recipe for a lavender and red wine butter which makes a steamed fish dish fit for a king!

red wine to taste
2 teaspoons dried lavender
3 shallots
parsley

salt and pepper
1 tablespoon balsamic vinegar
560 g (1¼ lb) unsalted butter (softened)

To prepare: Pour a little of the red wine into a saucepan and add the lavender, shallots and parsley. Boil until reduced to about two tablespoons of liquid. Add a teaspoon of salt, a good dash of pepper and the balsamic vinegar and again boil. Allow to cool slightly and pour into a food processor followed by the butter. The processor will at first turn this mixture into a red liquid and then gradually into a pink, workable paste. Remove in handfuls and shape into rolls like logs which can then be wrapped in clingfilm or foil and put in the freezer until required. The lavender and red wine butter is now ready to be sliced into pats which can be popped on top of the steamed fish when you are ready to serve.

Desserts

Lavender Junket Pots

According to Henry Phillips in his *History of Cultivated Vegetables* (1822), during the early nineteenth century desserts were regularly served at table arranged on a bed of lavender flowers. However, this summer delicacy, which has been a special favourite with East Anglian families for generations, incorporates the plant rather than just using it as a decoration. The pudding is both delicate in flavour and attractive to the eye. The addition of nasturtiums – another flower which has been eaten for centuries – to the junket pots gives an extra dimension to the colour and flavour. Serves 6.

750ml (1½ pints) milk
1 teaspoon lavender honey
4 sprigs lavender
350 ml (12 fl oz) double cream (optional)
5 teaspoons rennet
12 nasturtium flowers
icing sugar

To prepare: Pour the milk into a saucepan, add the lavender honey and sprigs and – stirring all the time to dissolve the honey – heat the mixture until it is just about to boil. Leave for a few minutes to cool slightly, at which point remove the lavender sprigs. Now stir in the rennet and pour the mixture into individual junket pots (or ramekin dishes). Allow these to set at room temperature before placing in the fridge to chill. Just before you are ready to serve, slice the nasturtium flowers thinly. Then top each of the set junkets with double cream (if to your taste) and add the nasturtiums. Finally, dust these delicious junkets with icing sugar and serve immediately.

Sorbet with Lavender Honey

This pudding was originally eaten by French peasants in the Roussillon region of France and was made from a mixture of very fresh goat's cheese and lavender honey. However, it can easily be adapted using *fromage frais* which is widely available in shops and supermarkets. Like the Lavender Junket Pots, this dessert should be made on the day it is to be served. Serves 6.

340 g (12 oz) *fromage frais* (not low fat)
250 ml (9 fl oz) water
115 g (4$^1/_2$ oz) caster sugar
juice of 1 lemon
6 tablespoons lavender honey

To prepare: Place into a mixing bowl the *fromage frais*, water, caster sugar and lemon juice and whisk together. Pour the mixture into a shallow bowl and place in a freezer. Every thirty minutes, take the bowl out and whisk the mixture to avoid the formation of large ice crystals. About thirty minutes before serving, remove the sorbet from the freezer to the fridge in order to let it soften slightly. When you are ready to bring it to the table, spoon the dessert into individual dishes and drizzle the honey generously over each portion. The sorbet can also be made by freezing in an ice cream maker, again adding the lavender honey when you are ready to serve.

Lavender Baked Custard

This dish can provide a wonderful talking point at the table, because although most people are familiar with baked custard and associate it with the traditional yellow colour, this version comes out of the oven a delightful shade of pale green! But the taste is unforgettably delicious.

450 ml (16 fl oz) single cream
1 bunch fresh or dried lavender
100 g (4 oz) caster sugar
3 eggs

To prepare: Mix the lavender flowers into the cream in a saucepan and gently heat for ten minutes to scald it. Allow the mixture to cook and then strain into a bowl. Add the caster sugar and beaten eggs and mix well. Pour into an ovenproof dish and bake in a moderate oven at Gas 5/190°C/375°F until you can see that the custard is set. Deliver to the table and wait for the cries of astonishment from your family or guests.

Lavender Ice Cream

For all those who love ice cream, this is a delicately scented variation with an unusual flavour that deliciously rounds off a three-course meal. It is believed to have been first developed in France, but I have chosen an English recipe which is certainly among the tastiest, and is from my home county of Suffolk. Serves 4.

4 egg yolks
75 g (3 oz) caster sugar
200 ml (6 fl oz) full-cream milk
100 g (4 oz) honey
200 ml (6 fl oz) double or whipping cream
6 fresh lavender flower-heads

To prepare: Cream the egg yolks with the sugar. Boil the milk and then pour this onto the yolk mix. Slowly cook until the mixture slightly thickens – be careful not to let it go lumpy. Mix together the honey and cream, and pour the egg mixture over. Infuse with the lavender flowers until you can tell by tasting that a nice flavour has been created. Then strain the ice cream and put in the freezer, stirring regularly until it is frozen. Alternatively you may care to use an ice cream maker if you have one. Lavender ice cream should be served with thin, crisp biscuits – perhaps even chocolate wafer biscuits if you have a really sweet tooth!

If you like finishing off a meal with cheese, crumble a few dried lavender flowers onto a piece of ricotta – this tip comes highly recommended from an Italian friend.

Afternoon Tea

I suggested several methods of making lavender tea at the start of this chapter, and individual taste will obviously dictate your choice for an afternoon cuppa. In the seventeenth century, many ladies took their tea with a spoonful of lavender sugar which was made by beating lavender flowers into three times their weight in sugar. Today, you may prefer to place two or three lavender heads in a sugar canister to give the sugar a lovely scented taste and aroma.

Lavender Jelly

My grandmother used to make this conserve with the lavender and cooking apples from her garden, and she often said that no afternoon tea was complete without a slice of bread and lavender jelly.

2.5 kg (6 lb) cooking apples
2 kg (5 lbs) sugar
5 tablespoons lemon juice
small teacup of fresh or dried lavender flowers

To prepare: First wash and prepare the apples. Chop them up, core, seeds, peel and all, and put into a pan. Boil gently – a tablespoon of water may be added at the start of the cooking process to prevent burning and help the fruit break down. Cook until they are pulpy (which should take about 30 minutes) and then pour into a jelly bag and leave to drain overnight into a bowl. Now you are ready to begin making the conserve. Measure out the apple juice and add 450 g (1 lb) of sugar to every 600 ml (1 pint) of juice. Pour this into a pan and add the lavender. Bring to the boil and allow to continue boiling for approximately 20 minutes, when the setting point will just about have been reached (105°C/222°F on a preserving thermometer). Skim off the surface scum and stir in the five tablespoons of lemon juice. Pour into warmed jars and seal carefully. When these jars are re-opened, the aroma of apples and lavender is like the fragrance of a summer day.

Lavender and Lemon Sponge Cake

The perfect conclusion to an afternoon tea – and one of the easiest to make. Although I have provided a popular sponge recipe in which the lavender can be utilised, do not hesitate to use your own favourite mix as this will work just as well.

100 g (4 oz) self-raising flour
1 teaspoon baking powder
100 g (4 oz) soft margarine
100 g (4 oz) caster sugar
2 eggs
2 teaspoons dried lavender flowers
1 dessertspoon lemon juice
grated rind of 1 lemon

To prepare: Sift the self-raising flour and baking powder into a mixing bowl, giving them plenty of air, and follow this by adding the margarine, sugar and eggs. Whisk with an electric hand-mixer. Fold in the dried lavender flowers, the lemon juice and the grated rind.

Continue until thoroughly mixed. Then divide into two 18 cm (7 in) sponge tins lightly greased and lined with greaseproof paper; bake for thirty minutes in the oven which has been pre-heated to Gas 3/160°C/325°F. To test for readiness, press the cakes lightly with a finger: they should spring back into shape. Turn out of the tins and, when cool, sandwich the two halves together with jam or fresh cream and dust with icing sugar.

As with all cooking, using lavender as an ingredient will demand a good deal of patience and experimentation in order to find the amounts which best suit your taste-buds and those of your family and guests. But a herb that has been proven for its taste and aroma for two thousand years still has a lot to offer the adventurous gourmet today. *Bon appétit!*

Chapter 10
A Key to Love and Beauty

Be in no doubt about it: lavender is sexy and there are lots of ways to use the plant to improve your looks, aid romance, and better your love life. This fact has been clear for centuries, to people in the know, and is now coming right back into fashion again. Indeed, it is not difficult to utilise a number of the qualities in lavender – its fragrance, conditioning and beautifying powers, for example – to unlock a fresh world of pleasure and perhaps even find a new love. And the evidence that we have from the past is a clear indication of just what lavender has to offer for the future.

In rural England, for example, women have for generations been in possession of a seductive little remedy, passed from mother to daughter, which is said to be able to arouse the romantic inclinations of any man when he returns home exhausted after a long day's work. It is an aphrodisiac known as 'Kissing Comfits' – little sweetmeats that combine sugar (for energy), nutmeg (for stimulation) and lavender (for romance). There are several variations on the formula for making the tasty little morsels which have a distinctly sensual flavour about them. My recipe comes from Kent where it is known to have been used for at least 200 years – although I have heard suggestions that 'comfits' were actually invented in France, as breath fresheners!

The ingredients you require for making 'Kissing Comfits' are several fresh blooms of lavender, an egg, some icing sugar, ground nutmeg and a couple of dozen cherry stones. It is as well to start your preparations with the stones because they must be crushed and then powdered before they can be used. Next cut off the lavender-heads into small, manageable pieces and dip them into a bowl of well-beaten egg white.

Roll them into balls and pop them into the icing sugar. Now, while they are still damp, roll them in the nutmeg and, finally, in the powdered cherry stones. The results are delicious – but they come with no guarantee from me that they will improve your sex life!

The Allure of Lavender

The association of lavender with the art of love goes back even farther than 'Kissing Comfits'. According to one of the oldest traditions, the flowers are said to be lucky for lovers because of their bluish colour and are classed under the star-sign of Mercury. In some places it is still considered essential for a bride to observe the custom of placing a lavender bag in her trousseau to ensure she has a happy marriage and will bear children.

An old superstition which I encountered when researching one of my earlier books, *A Dictionary of Omens and Superstitions* (1978), recommended any young man or woman who wanted to know what their true love would look like, to drink a brew of dried lavender flowers and thyme mixed with honey and wine just before going to bed. The concoction was to be sipped while still warm and would conjure up in dreams a picture of the lover-to-be. Girls suspicious that a man who came courting them might be more intent on sex than romance could, it was said, protect their innocence by carrying a lavender posy whenever they were in his company. This surprises me, for I would have imagined such a posy would be more of an *attraction* than a deterrent! The same source also says that lavender is supposed to ensure chastity.

In parts of East Anglia I have heard people claim that lavender is not just good for scenting a bedroom and keeping away unpleasant insects, but that a sprig of the plant placed under the mattress will keep the couple who sleep on it faithful to one another. An even more curious superstition from France maintains that putting some lavender in the shoes of a man or a woman with a wandering eye will keep the sinner on the straight and narrow.

The Water of Love

Probably one of the oldest and most effective accessories in a woman's armoury is lavender water, the fragrant, refreshing and *alluring* liquid which ladies have been dabbing on their bodies for centuries. While collecting information for this book I came across two old recipes for making lavender water which are interesting and instructive and deserve inclusion here. The first is taken from an anonymous volume, *The Toilet of Flora*, published circa 1790.

> If you would have speedily, without the trouble of distillation, a water impregnated with the flavour of Lavender, put two or three drops of Oil of Spike, a lump of Sugar, into a pint of clear Water, or Spirit of Wine, and shake them well together in a glass phial, with a narrow neck. This Water, though not distilled, is very fragrant.

The spike oil mentioned in this recipe has always been considered inferior to true lavender oil and was traditionally only used to dilute the more expensive oil because, despite its cheapness to produce, the quality was reliable. And even though it has a clean, fresh smell and has been used to scent detergents including liquid cleaners, soaps and shampoos – in some of which it actually replaced lavender oil altogether – spike lavender was never extensively cultivated and is now uncommon. The second recipe is from a wonderful volume entitled *Enquire Within Upon Everything*, which ran through literally hundreds of editions during the Victorian era. It reads as follows:

> *Lavender Water* – Essence of musk, four drachms; essence of ambergris, four drachms; oil of cinnamon, ten drops; English lavender, six drachms; oil of geranium, two drachms; spirit of wine, twenty ounces. To be all mixed together.

While both sets of instructions are probably workable, I think a few more practical instructions would assist the reader who wants to try making her own bottle of lavender water. It is easier to do so with ready-made lavender essential oil and a bottle of spring water. Obtain a large glass bottle, preferably green in colour. Fill this almost to the top with the spring water and add four drops of lavender oil. Shake the bottle vigorously for a couple of minutes and then store it in a cool, dry place. Ideally, give the bottle a shake three times a day to help the process along, and after about ten days the lavender water will be ready for use as a face rinse or body spray.

In earlier times lavender water was an essential part of many people's daily toilet because the washing facilities we now take for granted were nowhere near as commonplace as they are today. Those blends which contained alcohol were especially popular among folk in fashionable society because this meant the lavender water evaporated much more quickly and was ideal for cleansing the skin.

Lavender water has long been famous for use in hot weather as it cools and refreshes the body very quickly. But do not overlook its cosmetic properties and its ability to act as a long-lasting deodorant. It can also be sprinkled on clothes and linen after they have been washed, and may be applied at the ironing stage or when the items are being folded prior to putting away.

Days of Perfume and Lavender

For many years lavender was one of the main ingredients in smelling salts, which were so essential to Victorian ladies who were forever seemingly being overcome by emotion. (A more likely explanation was that they were suffering because their stays were too tight!) It was used in perfume, too (and still is), notably eau-de-cologne, which is a blending with alcohol of several essential oils, all known for their stimulating properties, such as bergamot, lemon, petitgrain, balm, rosemary and lavender.

Napoleon Bonaparte was a great believer in the powers of lavender, and is said never to have been without a bottle of his own personal eau de cologne made from a secret recipe which he named Eau Imperial. He told the members of his intimate circle of officers that he believed eau de cologne to be good for health, hygiene and morale. It has recently been suggested by a member of the French

Perfumer's Society, attempting to rediscover Napoleon's secret recipe, that the real reason for his extraordinary animal magnetism, and for his legendary ability to persuade troops to fight even in the harshest conditions, lay in this cologne which he splashed liberally on himself. He apparently also set great store by an aphrodisiac drink consisting of freshly brewed coffee, hot chocolate and musk water (mixed in equal parts) and drunk hot with several spoonfuls of lavender sugar. It seems he never missed consuming one of these before a night of love-making with Josephine!

The Gentleman's fragrance

Many male readers may be surprised to learn that lavender is a component in quite a number of the fragrances created especially for men. Because lavender combines well with a variety of other oils and helps to release their different qualities, the fact that it is there often goes unnoticed – a deliberate ploy by certain manufacturers apparently concerned that lavender's general association with female fragrances might deter some men from buying their products. To give any suspicious male who might be reading this an idea of what a lavender-based preparation smells and feels like, try the following recipe for a splash-on cologne which was recommended to me by a London perfumer and can be used on either the face or body. With vodka as one of the constituents, resistance to it may be that little bit easier to overcome!

The ingredients required are five drops each of lavender, bayleaf and bergamot oils; ten drops of petitgrain oil and 15 drops of oil of lime; 250 ml (8 fl oz) each of rosewater and vodka, plus two fresh limes and a teaspoon of benzoin tincture. (The benzoin acts as a preservative and an astringent and also has mild antiseptic qualities.) The first part of the procedure is to measure the vodka into a jar and then peel the limes and put the peel into the alcohol. Cover the jar and leave it in a cupboard for about a week. After this period of time has elapsed, take a second jar and mix in it the oils, benzoin and rosewater. Stir thoroughly. Now strain the vodka, throw away the peel, and mix the two liquids. Stir vigorously once more,

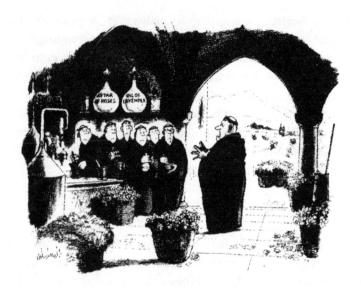

'The Church must move with the times, brothers – we're going into the after-shave business!' A topical cartoon by Thelwell (*Punch*, June 7, 1987).

bottle the liquid and leave it to mature for about four weeks. The resulting cologne should be strained though a paper filter before re-bottling once more. It is now ready for splash-off!

Beauty Potions

The women of Ancient Egypt were among the first to benefit from the beautifying properties of lavender, and there is evidence that it was used in a number of their cosmetics. In the intervening centuries we have discovered quite a lot about these preparations, and those used by women in other countries down the years, all of which has added to our knowledge of what the plant can do for our skins and complexions.

Experience has shown that lavender water is most suitable for delicate and sensitive skins – it is a great healer because it speeds up cell replacement and its mildly antiseptic properties help to reduce acne. Lavender oil, on the other hand, is good for virtually all types of skin – normal, dry, oily, sensitive and even mature and wrinkled. A good combination of oils which is recommended for all skin types except the very sensitive consists of four drops of lavender and two of geranium mixed with 20 ml (1 fl oz) of almond oil and 10 ml (½ fl oz) of jojoba.

An aromatherapist I know, who has treated a lot of young female clients suffering from acne, recommends the following blend as a curative: two drops each of lavender, tea tree and patchouli in 30 ml (1½ fl oz) of jojoba oil. I am told that a blend of 30 ml (1½ fl oz) of face oil should last for about a month and allow for an application three times per week.

In France many women have recently taken to applying a 'lavender oil mask' for cleansing and revitalising dry facial skin. It is not difficult to make up, and used just once a week will, it is claimed, noticeably improve the skin texture. You require two drops of sandalwood, one each of lavender and camomile and two teaspoons of honey (preferably lavender honey). After blending the oils with the honey, gently spread the mixture evenly all over your face. Keep the mask on until it no longer feels cool – usually two to three minutes – then rinse off and apply a moisturiser.

There is also a lavender moisturiser which you might like to consider making up. You will need lavender and almond oil plus a cup each of camomile and elder flowers. Simmer the two types of flowers in a little water for ten minutes and then add 20 drops of lavender and one teaspoon of almond and stir gently. Allow to cool. If the moisturiser is not thick enough, a little beeswax should be added while the liquid is still hot. The lavender moisturiser should be kept in a sealed jar in a cool spot. It is best applied last thing at night before going to sleep.

Fighting the flab

Cellulite, that curse of female beauty, which usually shows up as lumps on the thighs and buttocks and is believed to be caused by a build-up of fluid and toxins in the tissues, can be tackled by lavender oil because it is a diuretic and will help reduce fluid.

Although it would be quite wrong of me to claim that lavender is a wonder cure, because cellulite is notoriously difficult to get rid of, you might like to try massaging the affected areas with the following formula. To 30 ml (1½ fl oz) of safflower (which has good penetrative power as a carrier oil) add four drops of juniper berry (a detoxifier), four of rosemary (a cleanser), and three each of cypress (a good tonic for the circulation) and lavender. Apply twice daily with the palm of the hand and continue until, hopefully, you notice an improvement.

Fresh Breath

Bad breath can be as much of a turn-off as any skin complaint and here again lavender can come to the rescue with a mouth-wash in which vodka also plays a part. This remedy for halitosis – which is usually the result of digestive problems, bad teeth, or possibly smoking – was given to me by an American herbal expert who swore by it. The ingredients are 5 ml (1 teaspoon) each of lavender, peppermint, fennel, bergamot and tea tree oils mixed in a bottle with the same amount of vodka and shaken vigorously. This concentrate will make enough mouth-wash for several weeks. To use, add four drops to half a tumbler of warm water and gargle twice daily. **Do not swallow the mixture.**

Beautiful Hair

Attractive, shining hair is a vital part of sex appeal and a simple lavender shampoo can improve the lustre and strength of hair. It consists of a mixture of a mild baby shampoo to which are added four drops of lavender oil. Massage thoroughly into the scalp and then leave in the hair for a couple of minutes before rinsing carefully in warm water. The results can be very beneficial. Also, each morning, sprinkle a few drops of lavender water onto your brush or comb and run this through your hair. It will leave your whole head feeling good and your hair shiny and smelling fresh.

That Loving Feeling

Once a mutual attraction between two people has been established, romance can usually be helped to blossom in the right kind of environment, where both feel at ease and are able to express themselves and their emotions. A room in which an oil burner is wafting sensuous fragrances can help generate loving feelings, and I have heard a number of people speak highly of a mixture based on ylang ylang and lavender. What makes ylang ylang so good is its sweet floral essence, like a mixture of jasmine and almonds, and the addition of lavender seems to enhance its sensuous, feminine qualities.

There is probably no better precursor to love-making than a massage to soothe away anxiety and stimulate the body and senses. There are, of course, many books available on the art of body massage, so here I would merely like to give you a few tips on the importance of lavender in a massage.

The last thing you want to do when feeling in the mood is to have to stop and make up some massage oil. So I recommend preparing the following blend and storing it in a secure bottle until the appropriate moment. The amount is enough for two or three body massages, and as a general rule it is not advisable to make up much more than this, because essential oils do deteriorate when stored for any length of time.

My lavender massage oil consists of three drops of lavender blended with two drops each of sandalwood and juniper berry in 15 ml (3 teaspoons) of carrier oil. Almond is my favourite for the carrier oil, because it is nourishing to most skin types and contains vitamin E (an antioxidant) which keeps longer than most.

Before beginning the massage or even applying the oil to your partner's body, touching him or her with caring hands will transmit a feeling of love and concern. Apply the oil first to the palm of one of your hands and then rub them together gently in order to warm and distribute the liquid. When you start the massage, concentrate on using your whole palms rather than just the fingers, as this spreads the oil evenly and releases the fragrance more readily. Light, gliding strokes heighten the sensations – and it is only fair for partners to change roles at least once during a session as part of foreplay.

Finally, a word or two about sexual energy. Any lack of this is more likely to stem from an emotional rather than a physical cause – perhaps caused by stress of your own or tension between you and your partner. The massage described above can be a great help in these circumstances. Burning your favourite oil in a vaporiser placed in the vicinity of the bed can also help to calm and revitalise the body and spirit. Let lavender work its spell upon you not only in this area of your life, but in all the others I have described in this book. And to paraphrase that famous line in the movie Star Wars, 'May the fragrance be with you!'

PART 3

Further Reading and Suppliers

Books

Bremness, Lesley. *World of Herbs*, Ebury Press, London, 1990.

Chaytor, D. A. *A Taxonomic Study of the Genus Lavandula*, Linnean Society, 1937.

David, Elizabeth. *Summer Cooking*, Penguin Books, London, 1965.

Davis, Patricia. *Aromatherapy: An A – Z*, C. W. Daniel, 1988.

Dawes, Nigel and Harrold, Fiona. *Massage Cures*, Thorsons HarperCollins, 1990.

de Gingins-La Sarraz, Baron Frederic. *Natural History of the Lavender*, Herb Society of America, Boston, 1967.

Dorfler, Hans-Peter and Roselt, Gerhard. *Dictionary of Healing Plants*, Blandford Press, 1989.

Evelegh, Tessa. *Lavender*, Lorenz Books, 2001.

Farley, Kristine. *Lavender: Growing and Using Lavender for Fragrance, Mood and Body Care*, Silverleaf Press, 2007

Festing, Sally. *The Story of Lavender*, Heritage, Gloucester, 1989.

Fischer-Rizzi, Susanne. *Complete Aromatherapy Handbook*, Sterling Publishing, New York, 1990.

Forbes, Leslie. *A Table in Provence*, Penguin Books, London, 1990.

Grant, Belinda. *An A-Z of Natural Healthcare*, Optima Books, 1993.

Grant, Doris and Joice, Jean. *Food Combining for Health*, Thorsons HarperCollins, 1984.

Hemphill, John and Rosemary. *The Book of Herbs and Spices*, Omega Books, London, 1984.

Hills, Lawrence D. *Down to Earth Gardening*, Faber & Faber, London, 1967.

Howat, Polly. *Tales of Old Norfolk*, Countryside Books, Norwich, 1991.

Jekyll, Gertrude. *Home and Garden*, Longmans, London, 1900.

Jekyll, Gertrude. *Wood and Garden*, Longmans, London, 1899.

Lavabre, Marcel. *Aromatherapy Workbook*, Healing Arts Press, Vermont, 1990.

Lawless, Julia. *The Encyclopedia of Essential Oils*, Element Books, 1992.

Maury, Marguerite. *Marguerite Maury's Guide to Aromatherapy*, C. W. Daniel, 1989.

McIntosh, Charles. *The Book of the Garden*, William Blackwood, Edinburgh, 1855.

McNaughton, Virginia. *Lavender: The Grower's Guide*, Garden Art Press, 1999

Meunier, Christiane. *Lavandes et Lavandins*, Edisud, Paris, 1985.

Pinder, Polly. *Home Made*, Search Press, London, 1983.

Radford, Joan. *The Complete Book of Family Aromatherapy*, Foulsham, 1993.

Sellar, Wanda. *The Dictionary of Essential Oils*, C. W. Daniel, 1992.

Shipley, Sharon. *The Lavender Cookbook*, Running Press, USA, 2004.

Silvester, Hans. *The Lavender Country of Provence*, Thames & Hudson, London, 1996.

Stuart, David G. *The Kitchen Garden*, Robert Hale, London, 1984.

Thomas, S. *Massage for Common Ailments*, Sidgwick & Jackson, London, 1989.

Trattler, Ross. *Better Health Through Natural Healing*, Thorsons HarperCollins, 1984.

Vickers, Lois. *The Scented Lavender Book*, Bullfinch Press, Boston, 1991.

Wildwood, Christine. *Creative Aromatherapy*, Thorsons HarperCollins, 1993.

Wildwood, Christine. *Flower Remedies*, Element Books, 1991.

Magazine

The Lavender Bag, available from: www.thelavenders.org

Useful Addresses

Advice websites

Alan Titchmarch (gardening): www.alantitchmarsh.com
BBC Gardeners' World: www.gardenersworld.com
GardenSeeker.com (UK and USA): www.gardenseeker.com
The Gardening Register: gardeningregister.co.uk
Herb Expert (growing and cooking): www.herbexpert.co.uk

The Royal Horticultural Society: www.rhs.org.uk
What's Cooking America (recipes): whatscookingamerica.net

Lavender Plant Suppliers

Arne Herbs, Limeburn Nurseries, Limeburn Hill, Chew Magna,
    Bristol BS40 8QW, United Kingdom
Tel: 01275 333399
Email: arneherbs@aol.com
Web site: www.arneherbs.co.uk

The Herb Garden, Hall View Cottage, Hardstoft, Pilsley,
    Chesterfield, Derbyshire S45 8AH, United Kingdom.
Tel: 01246 854268.
Web site: www.theherbgarden.co.uk

Natalie Hodgson PYO Lavender Farm, Astley Abbotts, Bridgnorth,
    Shropshire WV16 4SW, United Kingdom
Tel: 01746 763122
Email: astleyabbots@angelfire.com

Jersey Lavender Limited, Rue du Pont Marquet, St Brelade, Jersey,
    Channel Islands, JE3 8DS, United Kingdom.
Tel: 01534 742933, Fax: 01534 745613.
Web site: www.jerseylavender.co.uk

Long Barn Growers and Distillers, The Old Sheep Fair,
    Bishops Sutton Road, Alresford SO24 9EJ, United Kingdom
Tel: 01962 738684
Email: barn@long-barn.co.uk
Web site: www.longbarn.co.uk

Norfolk Lavender, Caley Mill, Heacham, Norfolk PE31 7JE,
    United Kingdom.
Tel: 01485 570384
Email: orders@norfolk-lavender.co.uk
Web site: www.norfolk-lavender.co.uk

The Pembrokeshire Lavender Company, Broomylake Farm,
Tavernspite, Pembrokeshire SA34 0NU, United Kingdom
Tel: 01834 831521
Email: pembslavender@aol.com
Web site: www.pembrokeshirelavender.co.uk

Lavender Essential Oil Suppliers

G. Baldwin & Co. Herbs, 171–173 Walworth Road,
London SE17 1RW, United Kingdom.
Tel: 020 7703 5550, Fax: 020 7252 6264
Email: sales@baldwins.co.uk,
Web site: www.baldwins.co.uk

Butterbur and Sage Ltd., Aroma House, 7 Tessa Road, Reading,
RG1 8HH, United Kingdom.
Tel: 0118 9505100
Email: info@butterburandsage.com
Web site: www.butterburandsage.com

Natural Touch Ltd., 18 Test Valley Business Centre, Nursling,
Southampton, Hampshire, SO16 9JW, United Kingdom
Tel: 023 8086 0758, Fax: 023 8087 3451
Web site:www.naturaltoucharomatherapy.com

Neal's Yard Remedies, Peacemarsh, Gillingham, Dorset, SP8 4EU,
United Kingdom
Tel: 0845 262 3145
Email: nyrdirect@nealsyardremedies.com
Web site: www.nealsyardremedies.com

Shirley Price Aromatherapy Ltd., The Old Factory, 8 Hawley Road,
Hinckley, Leicestershire LE10 0PR, United Kingdom
Tel: 01455 615466, Fax: 01455 615054
Training and orderline: 01455 615436
Email: training@shirleypricearomatherapy.com
Web site: www.shirleypricearomatherapy.com

Trade association

British Essential Oils Association, 15 Exeter Mansions, Exeter Road,
  London NW2 3UG, United Kingdom
  Tel: 020 8450 3713, Fax: 020 8450 3917
  Email: secretariat@beoa.co.uk
  Web site: www.beoa.co.uk

Aromatherapy Courses

Essentials for Health, 2 Dukes Place, Marlow,
  Buckinghamshire SL7 2QH, United Kingdom
  Tel: 0845 108 0088 or 01628 476 100
  Email: enquiries@essentialsforhealth.co.uk
  Web site: www.essentialsforhealth.co.uk

Purple Flame Aromatherapy, St John's Spinney, Gun Hill,
  New Arley, Warwickshire, CV7 8HA, United Kingdom
  Tel: 01676 542 542, Fax: 01676 540 777
  Web site: www.purpleflame.co.uk

Canada
West Coast Aromatherapy, 120, 5421 10th Ave, Delta, BC,
  V4M 3T9 Canada
  Tel: 604-943-7476, Fax: 604-943-7307
  Web site: www.westcoastaromatherapy.com

Australia
Eclipse Living Essence, 4/32 Ardross Street, Applecross,
  Western Australia 6153
  Tel (08) 9316 4650, Mobile: 0411 725 870
  Email: enquiries@aromatherapyaustralia.com.au
  Web site: www.aromatherapyaustralia.com.au

Acknowledgements

The author would like to thank Pip Miller who has been generous in her help with information in the writing of this book and also for supplying several of the illustrations which so delightfully enliven its pages. I am also grateful to Dorothy Hall, Sally Cook, Jane Coates, Christine Lawrence, Ann Head and Henry Head for their help with the text. The staff at the London Library, as always, were kindness itself in helping me to locate books and magazines, as were those at the British Museum Newspaper Library in Colindale. I must also express my thanks to the following newspapers for allowing me to quote from their columns: *The Sunday Times, The Observer, Sunday Telegraph, Mail on Sunday, Sunday Mirror, The Times, Daily Mail* and the *East Anglian Daily Times*.